The Self-Care Solution

Merry Christmas, hun.

Love,
Alison
2018

The Self-Care Solution

A Modern Mother's Essential Guide to Health and Well-Being

Julie Burton

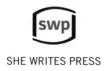

SHE WRITES PRESS

Published 2016
Printed in the United States of America
ISBN: 978-1-63152-068-6 pbk
ISBN: 978-1-63152-069-3 ebk
Library of Congress Control Number: 2015959045

For information, address:
She Writes Press
1563 Solano Ave #546
Berkeley, CA 94707
She Writes Press is a division of SparkPoint Studio, LLC.

Cover design © Leah Lococo
Author photo © Leslie Parker

All company and/or product names may be trade names, logos, trademarks, and/or registered trademarks and are the property of their respective owners.

Please note that suggestions in this book are not meant to replace the proper role of a psychologist, doctor, midwife, or other health-care provider. This book is not intended as a substitute for the medical advice of psychologists or physicians. The reader should regularly consult a licensed professional in matters relating to his/her health and particularly with respect to any symptoms that may require diagnosis or medical attention.

Dedication

THIS BOOK IS DEDICATED TO
DAVID, SOPHIE, JEREMY, ABE, AND JOSIE,
I LOVE YOU MORE THAN ANYTHING.
KEEP BELIEVING.

AND R.S., I REMEMBER.

Foreword

SELF-CARE HAS BECOME A BUZZWORD in this age of modern motherhood. For many of us, it feels like one more thing we need to do, and one more area of our overwhelming lives in which we feel that we are falling short. Not only have we failed to return the field trip permission slip on time, keep the house clean, and gracefully balance work and family, we're also failing to care for ourselves properly. Great!

In a 2015 keynote address in Denver, CO, Brian Smith, LCSW addressed a group of social workers, saying, "Self-care isn't an activity . . . Self-care is a *value*. . . We might even call it a superordinate value; care for that which embodies all the other values is too important to relegate to a throwaway cliché." I couldn't agree more. But motherhood in this day and age is already crammed full of to-do's; how can women realistically incorporate self-care into their lives? Most of them don't even know where to begin.

Julie Burton shows us where to start, and how to maintain an ongoing self-care practice in this much-needed, motivational book. Julie's balance of honesty, vulnerability, and practical advice found in *The Self-Care Solution* will profoundly impact the way mothers care for themselves as they care for their families. As co-editors of The HerStories Project and its four anthologies, we have read hundreds of women's stories about everything from postpartum depression to friendship to juggling work and new motherhood. We can definitively say, both in a professional capacity as editors and publishers, and personally as mothers of four children collectively, that there is a real need for this book.

Today's mothers are stretched to their breaking points. They are overwhelmed with trying to "have it all," and they struggle with the guilt that accompanies parenting in an era of competitive motherhood and too much information. They need help and reminders that, not only is it possible to take care of themselves, it is essential. *The Self-Care Solution* provides compelling evidence on the far-reaching positive effects of making self-care a priority, as well as the very real dangers of mothers neglecting themselves, their health, and their personal needs. Julie's genuine and empathic approach empowers moms to be intentional about self-care, and provides mothers with realistic solutions for overcoming self-care obstacles.

In addition to sharing her personal experiences as a mother of four, an eating disorder survivor, and a fitness and wellness instructor for the past two decades, she includes stories and advice from hundreds of mothers she interviewed. For mothers who want to better care for themselves but find that there are far too many reasons not to, *The Self-Care Solution* inspires mothers to move themselves up on that list, and provides comfort and guidance for mothers embarking on their essential self-care journey.

On behalf of mothers everywhere, thank you, Julie, for writing *The Self-Care Solution*. This book is a true gift.

—STEPHANIE SPRENGER & JESSICA SMOCK,
founders of The HerStories Project,
editors of *Mothering Through the Darkness:*
Women Open Up About the Postpartum Experience

Contents

Introduction

THE TEARS WELLED IN MY EYES, and I found myself shaking, sobbing, and struggling to catch my breath. But I couldn't stop running. I tried to run from the pain throbbing inside me. Though running had historically helped dissipate many of the worries and stresses within, this run was different. With each step, I felt my body and mind become more and more entangled with the swirling feelings of anxiety. Even as the sun warmed my skin and I willed myself to notice and be comforted by all the beautiful Minnesota summer greenery around me, I didn't feel better. My mind spun faster and faster, and the avalanche of cascading emotions made it impossible for me to separate them into manageable pieces. The racing thoughts moved from confusion to fear and began ferociously to seize my body—starting in my stomach, moving up into my chest, and lodging in the middle of my throat like a goiter-sized lump, making it hard for me to swallow or breathe.

I found myself in my sister's driveway, a few miles from my house, panting, gasping, reminding myself to breathe deeply, stop crying, pull myself together. But I couldn't this time. The floodgates had opened and I didn't have the strength to close them. I pounded on her door. I stood there, my legs shaking, my head bowed, snot running down my face, feeling desperately alone and afraid.

I heard the front door creak open and looked up to see my sister standing there, her eyes pooling with compassion and love. She opened the door and opened her arms as I fell into them. It took me a while before I could speak, before there was room between the sobs for words. But over the next few hours, I left a mess of tears and emotions splattered all over her sleeve and her living room floor.

When I had exhausted my words and tears, my sister simply looked at me square in the eyes and said, "You have to figure out a way to take care of yourself. You just have to, Julie."

Little did I know that, when I tied up my running shoes and pushed myself out my front door on that day in 2010—telling myself, as I often did, that I would feel better after a good run—the impetus for this book would be formed. I didn't know that on this particular run it would become apparent to me that I was desperately afraid—afraid that I was coming unglued, that I was losing myself, afraid that I wasn't the right person for the job entitled motherhood, that I was failing miserably. I was afraid that I wasn't equipped to handle everything on my plate: four kids, two of them challenging teenagers, plus a grade-schooler who had just been diagnosed with ADD, and a younger child who was a late bloomer and possibly in need of an extra year before starting kindergarten; a husband who traveled almost every week and worked late most nights; a father-in-law with a deadly cancer; other family and friends to care for; a recent financial calamity; family dysfunction; a friendship drama; a part-time job teaching group fitness; a desire to build my writing career. There was always more volunteer work to do in the community, and always more housework, more cooking, more driving, more errands, more homework assistance, more emotional supporting. How could I keep giving when I was running . . . out . . . of . . . steam?

This book grew out of a desperate plea to myself to figure out a way to take care of *me*, as I felt I was literally gasping for breath while being swallowed up in the sea of motherhood. My sister's message to me rang true, and yet I realized that I did not completely grasp what it meant to take care of myself and how I could put self-care into practice when so many people depended on me.

I realized, after breaking down to my sister, that while talking with family members and good friends about the nuts and bolts of motherhood had always been helpful, I often found myself too ashamed to reveal how overwhelmed and unsure of myself I had often felt. It seemed to me that every mom around me was mothering with way more ease and confidence than I was. But deep down I knew that this was not true, and that I was not alone in my struggles.

Rather than expose myself to people close to me (other than my sister), it felt safer to reach out to mothers whom I didn't know and who didn't know me. Utilizing my training as a journalist, I put on my investigative reporter hat and decided to pick the brains of as many mothers as I could in an effort to uncover all the coveted motherhood secrets that I had not yet been privy to—I needed to find out if I was missing something pivotal about the motherhood journey.

The mommy blogging phenomenon was not yet in full swing (or at least I had not tapped into it yet), but I utilized a motherhood website to post a twenty-two-question online survey about the trials and tribulations of motherhood.

The responses came in by the hundreds.

Ironically, my initial questions and book concept did not focus solely on self-care. I originally approached the writing of this book the same way I had been dealing with the stressors in my life. If I could just be a *better*, *smarter* and *more prepared* mother, then I would not experience the extreme levels of stress and anxiety that I had been feeling for some time. If I dissected, analyzed, and revealed every imaginable and unimaginable aspect of motherhood from birth to launch, I could prepare moms (myself included) for what lies ahead on their motherhood journey. So I took it upon myself to uncover the unspoken secrets of motherhood, and began to gather "the goods" from nearly four hundred moms who completed my online survey and the dozens I interviewed in person or via e-mail.

Through their experiences and my own, I decided, I would provide a tell-your-best-friend-after-a-bottle-of-wine, no-holds-barred portrayal of motherhood. By assimilating this information my readers would be protected from experiencing the extreme levels of stress and exhaustion that had nearly caused me to break down. My book would be a toolbox of sorts, where mothers could explore the various stages of motherhood and find management strategies for dealing with all of the ages and stages. Moms would be READY to tackle motherhood with confidence and grace! My book would start where Heidi Murkoff's *What to*

Expect series and Vicki Iovine's *The Girlfriends' Guide* books left us hanging.

Although I learned a lot from the plethora of good information I gathered—some of which is shared in this book, and which certainly has been used in my life—this book evolved into something very different as I went through the writing process. Along the way, I made a transformative connection that was pivotal for me in my journey as a mother and in the development of this book. I realized that obtaining knowledge about motherhood was not the key component of my being a happy and effective mother.

No matter how much of an "expert" I became on the various stages of motherhood, I still felt anxious as a mother. It wasn't until I dug deeper into the research, and moved past the tips on how to deal with tantrumming toddlers and teenage drama, that I started to see more clearly where my angst, and the angst of so many mothers, originates. My "aha moment," both for this book and for myself, occurred when I finally opened my eyes wide enough to see the most important question I had asked in my survey, and began to explore it with a therapist I had started seeing (a big step in practicing self-care). The question was, "How do you balance taking care of yourself while you are working to take care of your family?"

And there it was. The pattern was clear—I was indeed not alone. I found myself poring over the confessions of the hundreds of mothers who filled out my detailed, personal, "give it to me straight" survey until the wee hours of the morning. They shared their struggles, joys, epiphanies, and thoughtful advice about being a mother, about maintaining their relationships with their partners and their children, and about finding the balance between taking care of their own needs and caring for their families. Regardless of the varying demographics, family structures, work statuses, or numbers of children, virtually all moms surveyed (and I feel safe in saying that this sample speaks for the masses) feel that they are pulled in too many directions, habitually put others before themselves, and struggle to hang onto to some semblance of who they once were and, in many cases, who they want to be. Some, like the following two mothers, revealed that maintaining their sense of self was impossible. "I lost me, there is only Mom now, no time for Jane at all" (mother of two children, ages eleven and two). "Nurturing myself is non-existent. I put all my energy into my child" (mother of a two-year-old).

Although many of the women's stories were vastly different from mine (single moms, moms in abusive relationships, moms whose kids or spouses have health issues and/or special needs), I realized that I connected to almost all of them in obvious or subtle ways. I clung to their words, absorbed their advice, and felt grateful to each of them. I believe that—unbeknownst to them, and to me at the time—the honesty in their words helped reframe my situation, and provided me with a great deal of comfort that prevented me from spiraling further downward.

As I took an internal inventory of what I was and was not doing in the self-care department, I began to take comfort in the voices of the moms who are scattered on the pages of this book, who told me to let go of being perfect, to trust that I am doing the best that I can, to understand that I must take care of me as part of taking care of "them." I also felt sadness for the moms who admitted to neglecting themselves for the sake of their families, and I knew that I had to speak out to these moms and tell them that they have a right to feel good, to care for themselves, and to ask for help because they are worth it. In speaking to these moms, I am also reminding myself.

Veteran moms like these provided good reminders for me about why moms must take care of themselves:

> *As a stay-at-home mom I was able to hire some help*
> *a few mornings a week and I would work out or meet*
> *friends—I never wanted to resent my family . . . a*
> *happy Mom is key to a happy home!*
>
> —MOTHER OF TWO CHILDREN,
> *ages nineteen and seventeen*

*I had to learn to take good care of myself. For me,
regular workouts, even if it meant getting a sitter for
one hour. Also, time out with hubby and time out with
friends. I am a big believer in needing balance and that
a little time away from the kids makes for a happier,
better, refreshed Mommy.*

—MOTHER OF THREE CHILDREN,
ages nineteen, fifteen, and seven

*I take good care of myself. I've always maintained a
regular exercise program. I would never get pregnant
with another child until I had lost all the weight from
the previous child. I joined book groups and play groups
to make friends and stay connected with adults.*

—MOTHER OF FOUR BOYS,
ages eighteen, sixteen, fourteen, and nine

Throughout the process of reading, analyzing, and categorizing the survey responses, it became more and more clear that my breakdown did not occur because I was an ineffective or underprepared mother. No amount of preparation could have readied me for the unparalleled jolt I experienced when I felt the very first flutter in my stomach, signaling the new life within, a life that was mine, that I was responsible for, and whose survival was dependent on me—or when I saw my daughter's piercing blue eyes stare up at me for the first time. I don't know that any words of wisdom could have "enlightened" me about the overwhelming onslaught of new, raw, unstoppable emotions that swept into the depths of my soul, and sent messages to my brain each time I gave birth, that there never had been—and never would be—anything more important to me than the care and keeping of this child. And I most definitely could not have foreseen that the perfectionist in me would take over and slowly begin to tear relentlessly at my being. No amount of "motherhood preparedness" could have chased away the self-deprecating voices of those all-too-familiar gremlins perched on my shoulder speaking in loud, disparaging, and convincing voices: "You need to do *more* for your child. How *dare you* leave her? Are you sure you are doing everything *right*? How can you *not know* how to handle your child? Some kind of mother you are."

I also wasn't prepared for some of my childhood wounds to burst open unexpectedly as I mothered my four children. I didn't realize that a nearly insatiable need to heal these wounds would arise, which would propel me to set my own needs aside in an effort to make sure that my children would never feel alone or afraid in the way I sometimes had growing up. I couldn't predict that in mothering my children, I would begin a pattern of overcompensating for what I felt was missing for me as a child. Confronting your past and nurturing your whole self (past and present) while mothering your children is an integral component of self-care.

I have learned through research and throughout my own self-care journey that self-care is a choice, and that to be able to make that choice, the notion that "I am worthy of taking care of myself" needs to be deeply rooted in mothers. If they do not feel that way, then they would be best served to peel back some layers with a therapist, spiritual advisor, or trusted friend and discover where that message got lost, and how they can re-create it for themselves. Because no matter how hard one tries, if a mom does not *truly* believe that she deserves to take care of herself, the ongoing and forceful demands of motherhood will continue to derail her attempts to do so.

Those mothers who have stopped advocating for themselves and attending to their own needs—like the two women I quoted earlier in this introduction—seem defeated, as if they have lost a battle. I have learned firsthand that this is a battle mothers cannot afford to lose. I would challenge these mothers and plead with them as I had to plead with myself: stay connected with your sense of self, and of your self-worth. Remember who you are, separate from your child and your partner, so you can remain grounded and happy within yourself and be able to share your individual gifts with those you love. In writing this book I tracked my own self-care journey, and sorted through what worked and what didn't; this book offers guidance and encouragement for other mothers to track their own journeys.

A mother of a two-year-old and nine-month-old reiterates this essential message: "It has challenged me to constantly put others before me, at all costs. You need to nurture yourself so you can nurture your children. You need to hang onto your sense of self so you remember who you are, what you need, and what makes you happy—and then, and perhaps only then, can you give unreservedly to those who need you."

Breaking down the many such helpful suggestions into digestible pieces, while peeling back my own layers and discovering what self-care means to me in my life, crystallized the magnitude of my quest—to uncover the true meaning of self-care for moms, to validate the necessity of developing and maintaining an intentional self-care practice, and to provide tried and true methods for mothers to incorporate self-care into their everyday lives.

Throughout this book, you will discover that practicing self-care means setting clear boundaries, which sometimes means saying "no": *no* to being a room parent or being on a planning committee for a fundraising event (even though you feel that you really *should* do it and your good friend is begging you); *no* to taking on too much emotional baggage from an overly needy friend; *no* to taking on that extra project at work. And sometimes it means saying "yes": *yes* to any of the above-mentioned requests if they will be fulfilling to you or because you need the extra income; *yes* to a walk with a friend during lunch, even when you are on deadline for a project; or *yes* to taking a weekend trip away with your husband—even when you find out that you will be missing three of your son's swim meets, two of your daughter's basketball games, and your other daughter's first sweetheart dance (ask your best friend to take the pictures). Say yes to you. Say yes to what makes you happy.

My self-care journey included trusting my inner voice and having the confidence to speak it, while defining and maintaining my boundaries so that I could carve out the space I needed for me to feel whole.

This book, through real-life stories, illustrates the immeasurable benefits to mothers who do prioritize self-care, and the negative and far-reaching effects on mothers who neglect themselves physically, mentally, emotionally, and spiritually. Although there is no fail-safe prescription to combat this common pattern of neglect among mothers, the research and experience detailed on the following pages illuminates how self-care can truly be a matter of life and death. Not taking care of oneself can cause or trigger disease and dis-ease (anxiety, depression, addiction), or even death—not only in the morbid sense, but death to one's relationships and death to one's sense of self.

The *only* way that a mother can truly be present, engaged, connected, and nurturing with her child is if she is present, engaged, connected, and nurturing with herself. And the only way she can be connected with herself is if she does what she needs to do to care for herself in an honest and meaningful manner. This is the true essence of self-care for mothers.

This book is a roadmap for mothers to move toward self-care. No matter where you are on you journey, this book will help you to:

◆ Gain a clear understanding of what self-care actually means, and how and why it is directly correlated with being a healthy, joyful, connected, authentically present person, woman, mother, and partner.
◆ Identify efficient, manageable self-care strategies and practices that are the most effective, energizing, meaningful, or empowering for you and that can be efficiently integrated into your life.
◆ Identify barriers to self-care and solutions to overcome these barriers.
◆ Move you into action by shifting self-care from the back burner to the front burner.

Chapter 1:

My Life-or-Death
Journey to Self-Care

MY SELF-CARE JOURNEY HAS DEEP ROOTS. Unearthing these roots, and continuing to strengthen and secure them, has been, and continues to be, an integral part of this journey. It took me years to understand fully that, in order for me to practice self-care as a mother, I needed to go back to the pain: the pain that bumped up against the beautiful, magical, powerful love that filled my being as I birthed and mothered my children; the pain that accompanies a childhood trauma; the pain that resurfaces again and again as you realize that in mothering your children, you are also mothering and healing yourself; the pain that is diffused with large doses of love, and that reminds you that the development of your self-care voice begins long before you become a mother—and that *this self-care voice is about survival.*

Upon becoming a mother, I felt a volcano of overflowing love erupt inside my heart; but there were other unforeseen eruptions as well. I was no stranger to the feelings that spilled out on my sister's living room floor. I was no stranger to being afraid to ask for help for fear of being seen as a failure. I was no stranger to turning inward even when I desperately needed to reach out. I was no stranger to the perfectionism that led me to feel trapped and alone in my role as a mother and a partner. It took me many years to understand that *the mother's voice that reaches out and reveals her need for connection, love, support, and acceptance is the voice of self-care.*

MY TANGLED ROOTS

Putting others before myself was what I knew how to do. At some point during my formative years in the late 1960s and 1970s, while I was living with my parents and younger sister in St. Paul, Minnesota, I developed the notion that pleasing others (parents, coaches, anyone who would give me attention) was more important than caring for myself. I craved the acceptance and attention of others, and knew how to say and do things that people wanted or expected of me. I could adapt my persona to make sure the *other* person was happy and feeling good, even if I wasn't; and I grew to understand, through unspoken and spoken messages, that this was what I was supposed to do, and how I was supposed to act. In focusing my energies and attention on pleasing the "other," I neglected to develop a strong sense of self.

Much of my self-worth was determined by how others saw me, not by how I saw myself. I became adept at ignoring my own self-care voice. I did not fully understand how to communicate my needs to my parents and others, or how to advocate for myself to make sure those needs were getting met. I wanted and needed praise in order to feel whole, and didn't want to bother other people with my needs. Hiding many of my needs and feelings created a volcano-like feeling, which would erupt periodically in bursts of rage and extreme obstinacy. These behaviors both scared and confused me, and I began to distrust myself, disconnecting from myself and those around me. The volcano within was churning more and more every day, and at the age of sixteen, I could no longer contain the fire inside.

I had determined that not only were the external pressures too intense, but *I* was too much. I didn't like what I saw when I looked in the mirror—my outsides or my insides. My years of being a competitive gymnast had come to a close because the pressure (external and internal) became too much for me to handle. My muscular body was losing its form, becoming softer and curvier, and this depressed me. I began to feel socially insecure and to lose focus in school, and subsequently my grades began to decline. I told myself I didn't care—about any of it. But of course I did. I cared so much that it hurt, and yet I felt myself starting to give up, convincing myself that I could no longer fight the fight—that it was impossible for me to be all that I thought everyone wanted me to be, and all that I had grown to think I *should* be.

My conclusion, which I shared with no one, was that I was a failure, a sham, hideously imperfect and unworthy of love, care, or respect. The last straw occurred during a weekend spent at my grandparents' cabin the summer before my junior year of high school. A few friends and I had driven to the cabin, as did my older cousin and some of his friends. As we awaited my grandparents' arrival (they drove in separate cars), we received a call that my grandfather had been involved in a horrific car accident and suffered serious injuries. Instead of immediately going to see my grandfather in the hospital, none of us left the cabin. Without getting clear direction from our parents, we chose to stay for the weekend, acting like egocentric, self-serving teenagers.

Driving home, I felt nothing but shame and despair. Thankfully, my grandpa, whom I adored, was going to be okay, but I couldn't reconcile the fact that I had been so selfish, so inconsiderate, so *sixteen*. I pounded myself with "should haves" and "how dare yous?" "I should have left right away; how dare I spend the weekend at *his* cabin, lollygagging with my friends, while my beloved grandfather lay in a hospital bed fighting to recover? My family hates me. I hate me."

This incident provided the ultimate validation that that I was a horrible, unworthy human being, deserving of severe punishment. A riveting pain throbbed in my heart and in my head as the word "disappointment" flashed incessantly in my mind's eye. I desperately needed to numb the feelings of devastation, self-loathing, and rage toward myself and the world around me. With startling clarity and determination, I made a decision that it would be better if I disappeared—from myself and from the dysfunction in my family—and I turned a full-fledged firing squad onto myself.

Unbeknownst to my friends who sat sleepily in the car while

I methodically drove the sixty-mile stretch east on Highway 94 from Amery, Wisconsin, to St. Paul, Minnesota, I began a continuous-play mantra that would repeat over and over in my head long after arriving home—"I will never eat again. Never . . . ever . . . ever . . . " And for the next several years, I believed that this mantra would have the power and strength to drown out all of the other disparaging and paralyzing thoughts that lived like tapeworms within my being, eating away at my self-esteem and slowly, ever so slowly, eating away at my will to live.

My downward spiral of self-destruction and self-punishment manifested itself in a four-year battle with anorexia nervosa. My disease fed itself as I received a tremendous amount of initial praise and attention from family and friends for shedding the extra ten pounds I had acquired since quitting gymnastics. But red flags were missed or ignored, and the positive attention turned to concern and dread when I arrived home from a two-month study abroad program in Israel having lost another twenty pounds, one-fifth of my body weight. My clothes hung off my five-foot-one-inch frame. My cheeks were hollow and eyes vacant. I was depressed, terrified, and emaciated.

And for the next two years, I remained in the dark abyss of this brutal disease that included two hospitalizations, running away from home, and a stream of suicidal thoughts.

From an outsider's perspective, or so I have been told, it didn't add up. I had a seemingly "perfect" life within a seemingly perfect family. Most friends, family members, and acquaintances could not understand the whys and the hows of my disease. They couldn't grasp that the pressure cooker, which for years had been steaming within my family and myself, had exploded.

STRENGTHENING MY ROOTS

It took a huge amount of effort and many years to calm the fires within and tame this brutal disease. One step forward, seven steps back—taking accountability, denying, blaming, owning my truth, diverting, crying, raging, and trying, every now and then, to laugh. Admittedly, a good portion of my late teens and early twenties were spent in the trenches, with a brilliant, tough-as-nails, yet deeply compassionate therapist who helped me piece myself back together and find my way back to health. She helped provide me with the tools I needed to challenge my ongoing assertions that I was a colossal failure and to nudge myself gently onto the path that allowed me to fully grow into the person I am today. We looked at my family system under a microscope, and uncovered some of the answers to how and why I came to develop some of my "truths" about my relationship with myself and with the world around me. We peeled back my need for perfection, my fear of failure, my guilt, my shame, my regret, and my never-ending list of expectations—external and internal, real and perceived.

I rebuilt myself from the ground up, and as grueling and painful as this process was, I also found one of the most important elements to my recovery: hope. There were times when I wasn't sure I could do it, or even if I wanted to. I wasn't sure I had it in me to untangle the skewed ways of thinking and functioning that caused me to cling to the idea that I didn't deserve to be happy, nurtured, or loved. But slowly, deliberately, and sometimes terrifyingly, I began to break through my old patterns and formulate new ones—trading in feelings of self-criticism for self-acceptance, and self-sacrifice for self-care. Step by step, I slowly re-laid the foundation for my self-care voice.

Throughout this pivotal rebuilding process, for which I am eternally grateful, I found solid ground within myself, my family, and the world around me. And with that security, I simultaneously strengthened my mind and body, and my life began to move in a positive direction. I graduated from high school and college, achieved my goal of running a marathon (while maintaining a healthy weight), received a master's degree in journalism, secured a job at an advertising/public relations agency, and fell in love with and married my husband.

There were a multitude of bumps during those years, but I slowly allowed myself to trust those close to me and to reach out to friends and family for support when I encountered hurdles.

And even during times of struggle, the most critical lesson I had learned during my recovery changed the trajectory of my life forever: I would do everything in my power to make sure that *self-destruction will never again be my default setting.*

In disclosing the "ugly truths" of my past to my husband on our first date, I saw the fear in his eyes and the questions spinning in his head, some of which I asked myself. "Could this happen again? Will she be able to have children?" But I also saw his compassion. As our relationship deepened and trust grew, he would come to know that returning to that dark place was the last thing I wanted to do, and that I was committed to staying healthy in mind, body, and spirit. We were both committed to caring for ourselves and caring for each other. We worked well—as a team and as individuals. But nothing could prepare us for the life-altering changes and struggles we would undergo individually and collectively when, twenty-two months after we exchanged wedding vows, I became a mother.

CHAPTER 2:

Merging Motherhood with Self-Care

AS A SURVIVOR OF AN EATING DISORDER, I thought my newly strengthened and enlightened self-care voice was infallible. Years of going to therapy, and maintaining a healthy weight and a healthy attitude towards food and exercise, had brought me to a solid and secure place. I was certain that with a strong marriage, a good job, a network of friends, and a healthy lifestyle, I had this self-care thing *down*.

And I did—at least, at a time when I felt that I had control over my life, my decisions, and my relationships, and that I could manage what was on my plate. But at the age of twenty-seven, I could never have predicted how much more I would need to learn about self-care, and how challenging it would be to hold on to my sense of self, the moment I locked eyes with my newborn daughter's wanting and needing eyes. With goose bumps on my arms and my heart exploding with love for this child, I felt the "commitment for life" concept sink heavily and purposefully into the depths of my being. As I held her tightly in my arms, and took in the sight, smell, and feel of her, I promised her, and myself, that I would always protect her, love her, and care for her—that I would become a "baby whisperer," able to anticipate and accommodate her every need. I joined the ranks of mothers who have made similar statements:

I realized how wonderful life is. It is incredible to have something so small that I have never actually met before look at me for the first time and capture every single bit of my heart. To know love like that is amazing.

—MOTHER OF THREE CHILDREN,
ages eight, six and four

Motherhood has been the most amazing experience of my life; it has changed me in so many ways; enabled me to really love and connect with my children on so many levels, unlike any other relationship in my life.

—MOTHER OF THREE CHILDREN,
ages twenty, seventeen, and fourteen

When they handed my newborn son to me, I looked over my shoulder to see where the spotlight was coming from. There was no light. It just felt like there was. That was what amazed me the most about becoming a parent.

—MOTHER OF TWO CHILDREN,
ages twenty-two and eighteen

Like the moms above, I basked in the euphoria of my newfound sense of purpose and of the endless supply of powerful, all-consuming unconditional love that I didn't even know existed within me. I fell almost desperately, addictively in love with the feeling of being needed, revered, and loved by my daughter, and by my three subsequent children. And yet I didn't know that my motherhood journey would be twofold. Underneath this incredible, illuminating euphoria, there was something deeper—a residual, nagging anxiety that emerged from the scars within my heart, scars that had lain dormant since my recovery. Not until much later in my motherhood journey would I come to understand that the unresolved feelings that gnawed at me, wrestling with the joyous feelings of motherhood, were intricately connected to self-care; and that, as amazingly wonderful as motherhood often is, it is also really, really hard—

and that sometimes I was in way over my head.

It would be years until I fully grasped how my almost obsessive desire to protect my daughter and subsequent children was more than just a mama bear's "I want to keep you safe from harm" sort of quest. It definitely was that. But it also included an unspoken promise to protect them from the pain, the loneliness, and the despair that I had experienced as a child. And despite the fact that I put a lot of pressure on myself to "be there" for my children, in doing so, I continued to heal myself.

When my oldest daughter hit that ever-so-uncomfortable stage known as puberty, she began expressing some negativity toward the changes happening in her body. Initially, I was overcome with a sense of panic and dread. But quickly, I propelled my fear into a plan of action. The buck would stop here! I would take the lessons I had learned through my experience, through healing the wounds I'd endured while intently watching my mother fight her own food and body-image battles as I grew up. I would acknowledge my overwhelming responsibility to teach my daughter about all things related to body image, food, exercise, and nutrition. And after every discussion (and there were hundreds), I made sure she understood that all of the above-mentioned subjects are directly tied to self-love, self-respect, and self-compassion. I made a concerted effort to be a good role model for her in my approach to food and exercise, and kept the lines of communication open, checking in with her regularly to see how she felt about herself as she transitioned from girl to young woman.

I approached this issue with seriousness and intensity, practicing what I came to think of as a kind of double mothering, in which I cared for my daughter by reaching back deeply into my own childhood, providing love and compassion for both my daughter and my younger self. I held her when she cried as hormones surged through her confused preteen mind and body, and I gave her heavy doses of love, acceptance, guidance, and understanding during these trying years. I compassionately and gently helped her establish her foundation for healthy eating habits and body image in the way that

I would have wanted to learn them myself. And thankfully, at the age of twenty, she has one of the healthiest attitudes toward food and body image of anyone I know.

All three of my older children hit rough patches in middle school, difficulties that most kids cannot avoid as they are trying to figure out who they are, how they fit in, and who their *real* friends are, at the same time as they are pulling away from their parents. My kids experienced bullying, academic challenges, and self-esteem issues. As I write this book, in the fall of 2015, I am bracing myself for my youngest daughter's entry into middle school.

I worried tremendously about my kids during these trying years, as some of the pain of my own adolescence resurfaced. I did my best to give them as much love and attention as I could when they were struggling. But I also was very aware of the points at which I knew I needed to bring in outside support. Whether it was a school counselor, a tutor, a rabbi, a coach, a teacher, or a therapist, I did for them what I did not do for myself when I struggled: I asked for help. I knew I could not handle all of their challenges on my own, and I wanted them to feel that they were not alone in them—and that I wasn't either.

In mothering all four of my children through their various challenges, I have been able to mother different parts of the wounded child within me. My kids always know that I have their backs. They always know that they are not alone, and that I am able and willing to go down into the deep trenches of their lives and their psyches with them, in order to help them navigate life's inevitable twists and turns, as well as to help them develop a reflective, connected understanding and acceptance of themselves. They have learned that it is okay to ask for help, to trust in others, and to believe that there is a wide and strong net of people who care about them and who will catch them when they fall. And in doing that for them, I continued to trust that I could rely on the same reinforcements for myself.

However, because of my tendency toward extremes, and my deeply rooted "die on the sword" mentality, my "double mothering" would propel me in both positive and negative directions. It served as a constant push for me to become the best mother I could possibly be for my children and for the child within me, but it also provided a breeding ground of opportunities for me to be brutally hard on myself. While it was easy to feel good when the things I did to help my children worked out well, oftentimes my efforts did not yield the results I thought they would or should, or my children's behavior did not change at the speed at which I expected—as it goes with parenting. The old tapes containing messages of failure and disappointment played back in my head, sometimes even prompting me to look for "evidence" that I was indeed a failure as a mother. If my son got in trouble at school, well, guess whose fault that was? If my daughter didn't do well on a test, I should have helped her study more.

Needless to say, this critical self-care challenge caused me a great deal of angst and confusion before I understood that self-care lies far below the surface, in the place where our most wounded self resides. I realize now that my first decade of mothering provided me with a new platform for my embedded feelings of guilt and self-doubt, and my striving for unattainable perfection, to reappear. Slowly, subconsciously, and unintentionally, as my pattern would go, I began to slip away from who I was. I let go of many of my personal and professional goals, as many moms do (at least for a period of time), and I convinced myself that my only *real* purpose was to give to my family—until, years later, these feelings finally knocked me down and left me in a heap on my sister's living room floor.

Although I had worked diligently on solidifying my self-care voice throughout the process of my eating-disorder recovery, and was very grateful that I was even able to bear children (given the damage I had done to my body in my teens), I frequently felt alone, drained, unhappy, and unable to find solid ground. I did not yet realize that mothering them, obsessing about every little detail of their lives, would not bring me the fulfillment I needed to feel whole, nor would the idea that sacrificing my need to care for myself for "their sake" could be a healthy guiding principle for me, or for any mother.

The past two decades of being a mother and studying motherhood have taught me that I am most certainly not alone in this conundrum. Most mothers, while they nobly attempt to care for their children, struggle with defining their boundaries—which often leads mothers to neglect themselves. In a blog post on the website PsychCentral, journalist Margarita Tartakovsky explains why the mother-child relationship can feel so complicated. "Your relationship with your child isn't just symbiotic," she writes; "it's parasitic because it isn't a mutual relationship." She illustrates this point further by quoting psychotherapist Ashley Eder, LPC, who says, "Your children are—adorable [and] beloved— parasites, and you are the host, and that's normal and healthy." But in the spirit of self-care, the most important aspect of Eder's mother-child, host-parasite analogy is this: "The survival of a parasite is dependent upon the health of the host."

When a woman makes the transition to being a mother, and she feels the nurturing cells multiply by the second (or for some mothers who suffer from postpartum depression, it can be fear or even some resentment that kicks in), she is less inclined to be thinking about how to keep herself, "the host," healthy, and more likely to spend her energy on figuring out how to take care of her new "parasite." The following moms I interviewed echoed this sentiment as they spoke of their transition to motherhood and what surprised them the most about it.

> *I found it overwhelmingly anxiety-producing to think about the fact that we were 100 percent responsible for a helpless baby. And that life would never, ever be the same again.*
>
> —*MOTHER OF THREE CHILDREN,*
> *ages nine, seven, and four*

> *How very constant it is. And stressful. I feel like all I do is worry. I worry he will get sick or get hurt. I am constantly interrupted and feel as though I can never truly relax. I*

never realized it would change my life so much or change my relationship with my spouse like it has.

—MOTHER OF A SEVEN-YEAR-OLD

My life was no longer my own. I was, and still am, constantly preoccupied. I became a bit of a worrier. And the future suddenly took on tremendous importance. Everything got heavier. I went from being a relatively easygoing, almost passive person, to practically a warrior.

*—MOTHER OF TWO CHILDREN,
ages nine and seven*

As mothers like these admitted not only that the demands of motherhood were shocking to them, but also that they felt as if they had lost themselves and their drive to care for themselves as they cared for their children, my compassion and desire to help them avoid the following scenarios fueled the writing of this book.

Basically I take care of my son, then my husband, and have forgotten about myself.

—MOTHER OF A ONE-YEAR-OLD

At the moment, I do nothing to nurture myself. I need to start exercising and taking care of myself. I would love to make more real friendships.

*—MOTHER OF THREE CHILDREN,
ages nine, seven and four*

Someone always needs me, and my husband works odd hours, so I can't do anything regularly.

*—MOTHER OF TWO CHILDREN,
ages two and one*

While the moms above exemplify more of the extreme cases of losing oneself in motherhood, almost every mom I interviewed could connect with the feelings of frustration that often arise when talking about motherhood and self-care. In fact, if you pull a chair up to any table at Starbucks, an exercise class, park bench, set of bleachers, or office water cooler where a group of mothers are gathered and the topic of self-care comes up, you will hear many moans: "UGH, I just do not know how to do that anymore. Who's got the time?" "I have been trying to get to this exercise class for two weeks but my kids have been sick, my husband is out of town, and I am beyond exhausted. It is a miracle I am here!" There will be a unanimous consensus that finding ways to care for themselves while mothering children is one of the trickiest things they have ever done. They will compare notes on how much time and attention children demand, and then throw in their partners, work, friends, and other family members as other forces that tug at their energy.

For most moms, the idea of "self-care" can feel like just one more item to add to their already overflowing to-do list. And to some, like those quoted above, it can feel unattainable. For other moms, self-care practices will go in fits and starts. They will try. They will have intentions of taking good care of themselves, but will often get swept up in the needs of others and allow their own needs to fall by the wayside. They will express frustration, and sometimes even resentment: "I wish I had more time for myself but something/someone usually gets in the way. I was planning to go meet my girlfriends last night for dinner but Billy wanted me to stay home and help him with his homework. He didn't want his dad to help him, and even though I was angry about it, I stayed home to work with him. I feel so trapped."

In 2012, I attended a workshop for yoga teachers. One teacher, Megan, asked the workshop leader, Matt, a father of three children, including three-year-old twins and an eight-month-old, what we should do if we believe one of our students is battling depression. Megan went on to talk about one of her students who is a mom and is taking care of her young kids and her aging parents as well. The woman confided in Megan that she often felt resentful, anxious, and depressed because she was pulled in so many directions and felt completely tapped out.

Matt paused for a moment and replied, "It's like this." He grabbed a marker by one end and handed it to Megan, who took hold of the other end. But Matt did not let go of the marker. As Matt held on to one end of the marker and Megan the other, you could see the push-pull effect between them as they both grappled for the marker.

Then Matt said to Megan, "Maybe I don't really want to give you this marker and I would rather keep it for myself, but I am not sure how to do this because now you want and expect the marker that I offered you and I can't really take it back. But I realize I really need it." He explained how sometimes we give things (or parts of ourselves) to others even though we don't want to, and truly need to keep these pieces of ourselves intact. So we keep hanging on but feel like we "should" give it away. This can certainly provoke anxiety, and is a reality for many mothers who give of themselves to those who need them (children, partners, parents, bosses), but struggle to hold on to important pieces of themselves.

The fact is that it doesn't work to give away something that you desperately need for yourself. Mothers' limbs, hearts, and brains are constantly being pulled in various directions; think of Shel Silverstein's classic children's book *The Giving Tree*, which can be read as a parable of the self-destruction that comes to those who offer too much to others, while keeping nothing for themselves. But your trunk needs to remain steady and strong. You learn about your strengths and weaknesses as your children coerce, push, and challenge you. The only thing you are truly in control of is yourself. By taking care of yourself mentally, physically, emotionally, and spiritually, you are more likely to be able to be strong for yourself and your kids and to be able to withstand the storms that come through your life and their lives.

ALLOW YOURSELF TO BE OPEN
TO SELF-CARE OPPORTUNITIES

During the four and half years between my second and third child, I had my first of several self-care wake-up calls. I was stuck in a spiral of questioning whether or not I even liked being a full-time, stay-at-home mom, especially with my husband traveling so often for work, and yet feeling uncertain what I wanted to do with my life outside of mothering my children. To top it off, I felt guilty for even "complaining" about these issues because I knew I was lucky to have the choice to stay home with my children. Nonetheless, I realized that if I did not incorporate some real, meaningful self-care tactics into my life, I was at risk of digging myself into a dark hole, a task for which I had already taken the shovels out. There would be other times over the years when I would lose my self-care way, but after many steps forward and many steps back, I realized that sometimes practicing self-care involves stepping out of your comfort zone and being open to ways to rejuvenate yourself.

This particular self-care "aha" moment occurred unexpectedly, when I allowed myself to take a break from my colicky baby. I had hired a babysitter so I could escape his crying for a few hours. I debated between going somewhere to sleep (which certainly would have been an act of self-care) but chose instead to take a spinning (group cycling) class at the local gym. Halfway through the class, I found myself exhausted and yet exhilarated. I felt the endorphins kick in and I felt alive in a way that I had not felt in some time. Tears streamed down my face as the teacher repeated the words in a gentle encouraging tone, "No matter what obstacle is holding you back, or causing you pain or sorrow in your life, you can overcome it. You have to believe that you can do this. You can get through anything if you believe in yourself."

As I conjured up the strength in my legs to push the bike pedals around and around, and sweat and tears flowed out of my pores and my eyes, I felt a powerful shift within me. In that moment of heightened emotion, I realized that I was powerless over my son's crying, for which I, of course, had blamed myself. I understood with a clarity that I had not experienced before that his colic was not my fault, that it was not a piece of "evidence" demonstrating that I was a failure of a mother. And I realized something else equally powerful, that I would get through my son's colic—even the darkest days, the ones when I thought that I couldn't make it through another hour. My son would not scream bloody murder for the rest of his life. *I would get through it.*

This thought filled my entire mind and body with hope. And lastly, I realized that come hell or high water, I would get a babysitter once a week and take this spinning class. Because I loved it. Because it made me feel like myself again. Because as challenging as it was, it felt good and it filled me with a happiness that I knew I had been missing. It connected me with myself in a way that I had let go.

And it didn't stop there. Not only did I realize how much I benefited from participating in group fitness, but I also realized that teaching group fitness, like I had done in my early twenties, was something that I badly missed. So, after much back and forth of questioning and doubting myself, I told my husband that I was signing up for spinning teacher training. Within six months, I was on a spinning bike, in front of a class of sixty spinners, blasting Michael Jackson, Journey, Bruce Springsteen, and Marvin Gaye, telling my students to tap into the inner strength and belief in themselves that would guide them through their challenges both on and off of the spinning bike.

By taking more risks like this, which sometimes seemed like impossible mountains to climb, I came to understand the importance of merging self-care with motherhood. I also understood that it would never be easy.

My twenty-year motherhood journey has led me to this present moment. I have a husband of twenty-two years and I have four healthy, well-adjusted (on most days) children—one in beginning her third year of college, one who is heading off to college, one who will be in his last year of middle school, and one who will be in her first year of middle school. As I juggle my parental duties with teaching yoga, writing, and actively serving my community, I have realized that there are three absolutes in my life as a mother and a wife:

1. **Someone will always need me.**
2. **No one is going to hand over the time and space I need to take care of myself.**
3. **I need to be intentional about caring for myself or I am not able to take care of my family the way I want to.**

IGNITE THE URGE TO MERGE

And then there are the moms, whom I have studied in awe (and admittedly with some envy as well), who figure out very early on that self-care is the key ingredient to feeling balanced, contented, and fulfilled in their role as mother and partner. These mothers reveal that they are intentional about taking care of their physical, emotional, and spiritual needs, and are therefore able to mother their children with positive energy and without resentment. They express a clear determination and commitment to making sure that they do something positive, restorative, and healthy for themselves on a regular basis. And the most powerful admission these mothers make is that they are *happy*. This is what self-care looks like for some of these moms:

> *Between a moms' group once a week, girls' night out once a month, meetings for my nonprofit, and purposeful alone time I do pretty well with recharging my batteries. Two years in a row, I took a vacation without my family—once with my dad to climb mountains and another alone to visit the ocean. Next year I'm planning a road trip with some girlfriends and possible mountain climbing. Me time is a must, and my husband completely understands. He even takes vacation time to be with the boys. He can tell when I need a break of more than just a night out. This makes*

*for a happy mommy that can handle the day-to-day
adventures more easily!*

　　—MOTHER OF TWO CHILDREN, *ages seven and five*

*I meditate, I practice yoga, I walk, I cook. I see a
therapist and I travel as often as I can.*

　　—MOTHER OF TWO CHILDREN, *ages ten and eight*

*I took an exercise class every Monday and Wednesday
afternoon. My kids knew it, my husband knew it; this
was 'my thing.' They all understood very early on that
this was pretty much sacred time to me, and that I
needed this to feel good so that I could be good to all of
them. Not much got in the way of this for nearly twenty
years. My kids are out of the house now but that class is
still part of my routine and is what helps me to feel good
physically and mentally.*

　　　　—MOTHER OF THREE GROWN CHILDREN

*I am starting to realize that I need to develop a sense
of myself if I am going to be a good parent for them. So
when I am unable to see them (i.e., they are with their
dad), I go out with friends, exercise, and try to relax. I
feel that this break allows me to appreciate them even
more when they return.*

　　　　—MOTHER OF THREE CHILDREN,
　　　　ages three and one (twins)

Other mothers, who are on much more limited budgets, revealed
that they are able to properly care for themselves without
spending a dime. These mothers "run every day on my lunch
hour from work," "soak in the tub after the kids go to sleep," or
"go for a walk every Saturday with my best friend."

Even mothers who claim to have a decent handle on their
self-care admit to encountering times when unpredictable
situations like illness arise and derail their plans. But in talking

to these mothers, I have concluded that another key ingredient to a successful self-care plan is resilience. While these mothers may have had lapses of time when they couldn't practice all of their self-care tactics, they expressed flexibility and the ability to stick with their overall self-care intention, even when they face obstacles. If they can't get to the gym because a kid is sick, they will walk up and down the stairs in their house when their baby naps. They do the best they can to incorporate simple, doable, effective practices, like taking a few minutes to meditate every morning or talking regularly on the phone to a friend who makes them smile. These seemingly small and insignificant acts are sometimes enough to carry moms through tough times, keeping them feeling grounded and cared for—and, for the most part, happy, even when life throws out its inevitable curveballs.

Throughout the process of writing this book, it has become clearer to me what self-care is and what it isn't, and that most moms linger somewhere between being completely disconnected from their needs and being Johnny-on-the-spot for meeting all of their needs (which, of course, is impossible). Most mothers are *trying* to be intentional about self-care. And trying is a great place to start. For those mothers who barely have self-care on their radar, congratulations—you picked up and are reading this book, which means that even though you may not have a self-care practice in place, you do believe that you have a right or even a responsibility to attend to your needs. Wherever you are in your self-care journey, please do not judge yourself harshly, since I truly believe that all moms are doing the very best they can. But I am here to say, as one who has hit rock bottom in the self-care department, that your life can and will get better as you begin to care for yourself in a way that you truly deserve.

As we visit the cornerstones of self-care over the course of this book, keep in mind that this concept is a marathon, not a sprint. While mothering, self-caring, and running a marathon may sound grueling and exhausting, the essential message is that while your self-care plan may be challenging to create and follow, it needs to be approached in a slow and steady manner. After all, it really is about the one-day-at-a-time journey on the path to feeling good, and there is no final "you made it" destination.

Self-care is not a mad dash to a virtual finish line; it is about meeting yourself where you are right now and constructing a plan that you can follow with kindness, patience, flexibility, and compassion. On your journey, there will be times when you feel like you've "got it"—you're in your groove—and there will be other times when you feel like your plan is not working the way you had hoped, that it is way harder than you thought it would be, and that you want to throw in the towel. But like anything in life, as you encounter the inevitable tough spots, you need to reach out to your support system for help, and look for the strength inside yourself. And always keep in mind that you are on a powerful, potentially life-changing journey that will open up new pathways in your mind, body, spirit, and relationships with others—pathways that you may not have even imagined to be possible.

REMEMBER—YOU ARE IN CHARGE

"Signing up" for motherhood certainly does include a never-ending spreadsheet of responsibilities. Moms often feel that they walk around wearing a uniform, just waiting to put out the next "fire" (whether it be a child's friendship misunderstanding or a broken heart), or to chauffeur a child to the next play date or baseball practice, or to race to pick up a husband's forgotten dry cleaning. However, the most essential message that mothers need to tell themselves, even during firestorms, is this:

You are in the driver's seat of your life. You are in charge of the way you take care of yourself physically, mentally, emotionally and relationally. No one else, not your child or your spouse, determines if or how you take care of yourself.

Motherhood can be one of the richest, most fulfilling, and most amazing aspects of your life, *especially* if you continue to foster *you*—your passions, desires, hopes, and dreams. While moms may need to do some internal and external adjusting and rearranging in terms of the timing of when and how they manage their life's fulfillment, there is no need to turn yourself into a sacrificial lamb for your children.

The single best thing I have done as a mother, for my family and for myself, has been my continual work on strengthening my self-care voice. And unbeknownst to me in my early days of becoming a mother, doing so was so much more than taming that punitive, self-critical voice that once told me that I would never eat again because I was worthless. Though I made the conscious choice not to use food as a vice twenty-five years ago, in the same way a recovering alcoholic makes the decision to abstain from drinking, the path to healing and to true, lasting self-care in both cases goes far beyond changing those behaviors themselves. Whether or not they have suffered from an addiction, most people do develop some negative thought patterns, old tapes replayed in their heads, that can be destructive and can work to pull them away from their true selves. Because as a mother you have such a critical role in nurturing your family, it is crucial that you continue to challenge any internal (or external) negativity about yourself, and to incorporate two essential elements of self-care—self-love and self-compassion.

While using self-love and self-acceptance as your guides, the following tools, which will be detailed in the following chapters, are the critical components to successfully merging motherhood and self-care:

- ◆ Move your body, nourish your body, and rest your body.
- ◆ Stimulate your mind and activate your spirit.
- ◆ Nurture your relationships (with your partner, your children, your family, your friends, and yourself).
- ◆ Establish healthy boundaries.
- ◆ Connect with and heal your inner child.
- ◆ Be gentle and compassionate with yourself and others.
- ◆ Find joy and gratitude in every day.

CHAPTER 3:

Self-Care Solution #1 — Honor Your Body

When I talk about physical self-care, women often assume that I am referring to the number of workout hours they clock at the gym or the number of green vegetables they consume in a week—an assumption that can immediately grab hold of a mom's hand and lead her quietly to the closest shame pit. So let's be clear from the get-go: as we talk about food, body image, and exercise (hot buttons for almost all women), my hope is to steer you as far as humanly possible away from any feeling that even relates to shame, because—as the most influential shame and self-compassion researchers, such as Brené Brown and Kristin Neff, will tell you—shame is a direct hindrance to self-compassion. My hope is that when you think about the physical aspects of self-care, you will approach them from a place of self-love and compassion. As Brown explains in her book *I Thought It Was Just Me (but It Isn't): Making the Journey from "What Will People Think?" to "I Am Enough,"* "Shame corrodes the very part of us that believes we are capable of change."[1]

Shame may also correlate with the fact that so many women spend an inordinate amount of time thinking, obsessively and compulsively, about food and their bodies. A recent survey found that 67 percent of women in the US worry regularly about their appearance—more often than they worry about finances, health, relationships, or professional success.[2] And up to twenty million American women will suffer from eating disorders at some point during their lives.[3] We certainly have an uphill battle in this area of self-care. And these difficulties start when we are young, which is why it is so important for mothers to be extremely aware of the messages they are sending to their children. A study at Pepperdine University, published in the journal *Sex Roles* in October, 2010, shows that girls as young as three years old already aspire to be thin,[4] and separate research indicates that some are dieting by the age of six.[5] Unless you plan to hide under a rock to avoid television, radio, billboards, and all social media, it is impossible to escape the unfortunate reality that women's bodies are objectified and under constant scrutiny by society as a whole.

While many girls and young women struggle with body image issues well before they become mothers, these struggles often escalate after the inevitable body changes that occur during and after pregnancy. Many mothers continue to express frustration with their postpartum bodies, which they describe as "gross," "disgusting," and "saggy." Their ongoing self-criticism can negatively affect their self-esteem and the levels of happiness and fulfillment in their relationships, as well as the messages they pass on to their children. The ability to accept, embrace, and nurture one's body is a critical component to practicing self-care.

How refreshing it was to hear actress Jennifer Garner reveal on *The Ellen DeGeneres Show* in October 2014: "I asked around, and apparently I have a baby bump. And I am here to tell you that I do." The audience applauded, and Garner commanded them to "hold up." She continued, "I am not pregnant." The audience laughed. "But I have had three kids and there is a bump. From now on, ladies, I will have a bump. And it will be my baby bump. And let's all settle in and get used to it. It's not going anywhere. Its name is Violet, Sam, and Sera."

We need more Jennifer Garners out there delivering messages to women and mothers about finding love and acceptance of their bodies. No matter where you are, or where you would like to be, in regards to your weight or your view of your body, losing any amount of shame and self-loathing is the crucial first step toward acquiring a healthy approach to food and your body.

HOW TO WIN THE FOOD AND EXERCISE BATTLE

Spending time in the dark, lonely trenches of an eating disorder has given me a heightened awareness of the importance of dealing with the underlying issues that can cause women to obsess over food, and over their bodies, to mask feelings of insecurity and self-loathing. I have also witnessed firsthand—in my work as a fitness instructor, as a facilitator of parent support groups at the Emily Program (a treatment center for children and teens battling eating disorders), and as a mother—that if not approached in a healthy way, food and exercise can become dangerous addictions. There are now forms of food disorders that did not exist (or, at least, did not have a specific label) when I battled anorexia. *Orthorexia* is when one's obsession is not on how much or little one eats, but on how virtuous and healthful one perceives one's food to be; *exercise bulimia* is similar to bulimia, but instead of purging food, exercise bulimics over-exercise to burn the calories they consume.

Through my work at the Emily Program, I have come to learn more about the recent food- and exercise-related diagnoses. But no matter what label is attached to a particular food or exercise fixation or compulsion, the one certainty is that, if not approached in a gentle, self-compassionate manner, the management of one's diet can be a full time, all-consuming obsession, ultimately hindering your ability to be fully present, engaged, and connected to yourself and the people around you.

Throughout my disease and even during many years of my recovery, I did a great deal of experimenting with food and exercise, trying to find the "perfect" balance for me. It took many years to figure out what "normal" and healthy eating and exercising looked and felt like. As I look back, I can see that some of my experimentation was still tied to my desire to maintain a sense of control, not just of my weight but of my emotions as well. Focusing too much on food and exercise was still a way to prevent myself from experiencing my feelings and fully engaging in my life.

My food and exercise battle continued, and I experienced yo-yo weight gain and loss for some years after recovery. But as I continued therapy and gained a deeper understanding of myself and what it truly meant to listen to and respect the signs and signals of my body, I leveled out at a healthy weight. And then of course I was pregnant on and off for a decade, and while I loved being pregnant and basked in the feeling of freedom to eat what I wanted and in the knowledge that I was not only nourishing myself but my child, it was sometimes challenging for me to see my body change in unforeseen ways.

Between pregnancies, and after having my fourth child, I was easily swayed into adopting different food approaches. My kids went gluten- and dairy-free because of allergies, so I also went gluten- and dairy-free. A good friend became vegetarian, so yep, I tried that too, and then moved into a vegan phase. There were the low-fat, no-sugar, and high-protein phases. And while they were not "official" diets—like the grapefruit and egg diet that was in vogue during the 1970s—when I noticed my mother experimenting with various diets, they were restrictive nonetheless. While I learned a tremendous amount about food and nutrition during this experimental period, I knew this was risky territory for me. I tried to be honest with myself about my level of obsessiveness around different food plans, and eventually I would be able to ask myself if these phases were more about fear and control than about (for example) not wanting to eat an animal, or the fact that eating dairy does give me a stomachache. Noticing the concerned, "here we go again" look of family members as I passed on the turkey at Thanksgiving (because I was now a vegetarian) gave me pause, and forced me to closely examine my motives.

As I pulled away from this type of more restrictive eating, I realized that—even though my weight was healthy and I did not feel that I was in danger of slipping back into the disease—I was still battling some fears and insecurities, which manifested themselves in my desire to find control with food. Thankfully, I continued to peel back more layers, both through my work in therapy and by being honest with my husband and trusted friends and family members. I noticed that the healthier and more secure I became, mentally and emotionally, the more my relationships with food and my body followed suit.

As for exercise, it was much of the same. I ran thirty to forty miles a week for two decades, once completing a marathon in less than four hours; I trained for and participated in a biathlon and a triathlon; climbed thirteen thousand feet to the top of Pikes Peak to raise money for cancer research; taught high-impact aerobics classes, group cycling classes, Pilates classes, and yoga-sculpt classes—and now I teach restorative yoga to a high school girls' hockey team. Slogans like "Just Do It" and "What Doesn't Kill You Makes You Stronger" have required some tweaking in my brain over the years, as a strained hamstring from too much spinning—and the discovery in 2012 that I have degenerative discs in my back and neck—forced me to change many of my exercise habits. As much as I loved these high-intensity "killer" workouts (and still miss them today), I knew that I needed to turn up the volume on my self-love and self-compassion voices, which were begging me to slow down.

After my years and years of food and exercise experimentation, one word really has been the key to my ability to maintain a healthy weight without being that obsessive, crazy person whom you don't want to sit by at a restaurant because she is no fun around food and takes way too long to order—or the one who is such a slave to her two high-intensity workout classes a day that she only has thirty minutes to meet you for a raw juice between them.

That word is *moderation*. Moderation, in the truest sense of the word, is the first ingredient to finding your way to a healthy weight and to feeling good about yourself physically and emotionally. A punitive, restrictive, fast and furious, quick-fix approach to food and exercise is not your ticket out of food and weight battles or to maintaining the integrity and health of your body long term. "Research shows that, in general, people that diet still weigh more than their peers," reported Alison E. Field,[6] an assistant professor of pediatrics at Children's Hospital Boston; she found that mothers who overemphasize their concerns about body weight are significantly more likely to pass on these attitudes to their children.

The second key ingredient in your effort to steer clear of exercise, food, and body-image wars, and to maintain a positive self-care approach, is to focus on staying grounded in *gratitude* as you approach food and exercise. This sense of grounding (which will be discussed more in subsequent chapters) is derived from your underlying mindset about your body and the food you put into it.

It is essential to stay connected to gratitude—for the food you eat every day, and for the fact that you have access to abundant amounts of safe and healthy foods. Furthermore, if you can think of your body as something you are grateful for and something that is worthy of honor and respect, it is easier to understand the importance of treating your body well, filling it up with good nourishment, and making sure that you move it regularly so that it does not atrophy.

Being mindful of gratitude and worthiness is also very helpful for moms, like those mentioned in the previous chapter, who have no time or space in their lives to take care of themselves, as well as for all moms who deal with the general challenge of making their own needs as much of a priority as their spouses' and children's needs. According to Brené Brown, "Part of the process of cultivating worthiness is through self-compassion—treating ourselves the way we treat other people we love and respect."[7] We'll delve even more deeply into the benefits of practicing gratitude in chapter 5.

YOU ARE WORTH IT!

Over the past twenty years, as I've taught a wide variety of fitness classes to thousands of moms with a wide variety of fitness and wellness goals, many of them have shared their success stories with me. Let me clarify: when I talk about *success* in terms of exercise, I do not necessarily mean that these moms lost weight, although many of them did. "Success" to me, and to many of the moms I have worked with, means that they found a place of self-love and acceptance with their bodies. They felt better about themselves and they found joy in moving and strengthening their bodies, and in turn, their bodies often did change over time. While these women approached their exercise regimens with diligence and a committed determination, they also found a renewed connection with their bodies, minds, and spirits that helped to sustain their commitment on a deeper level. They showed up regularly to class with sincerely rooted (if sometimes reluctant) smiles on their faces, even if they initially struggled to keep up or to find immediate happiness in their new challenge. Their positive demeanor was twofold: they felt good because the exercise gave them an endorphin boost, and they also felt empowered by the knowledge that they were doing something good for themselves and their bodies.

The key elements that perpetuated my students' commitment, and kept them coming back for more, were their belief in themselves and their "I am worth it" attitude. And every single time they stepped back into class, I tried to validate those beliefs. I encouraged them to find joy and to feel grounded and connected by reminding them, "These next sixty minutes are a gift to you. No matter what is going on in your life, no matter how much stress you are under, or how many people are pulling at you and your time, this is *your* time. Cherish it and make the most of it, whatever that means for you today. You are making this commitment to your health because you are worth it. Do this for yourself. And you will be better able to serve yourself and those who need you."

Even those who did not stay committed to my class would excitedly tell me, when I ran into them outside the studio, that since attending my class they had checked out Jazzercise and kickboxing classes and decided that Jazzercise was "it" for them.

Bingo! I could see the twinkle in their eyes that was ignited by the feeling of empowerment and joy. They were empowered that they were embarking on a healthy path, and that they were being intentional about positively impacting their mind, body, and spirit. And they were having fun! This type of path was not only adding happiness to their lives, but helping them to be more positive, balanced, calm and connected people and mothers. In turn, moms are able to share this happiness and balance with their children and their partners. "Working out is my therapy," one mom of two children, ages fourteen and thirteen, explained. "I need that time to blow off steam so I am happier and less irritable with my kids and husband."

FIND SOMETHING THAT WORKS FOR YOU, AND JUST SHOW UP

Actor-director Woody Allen claims, "Eighty percent of success is showing up." In that spirit, I always start my fitness classes by congratulating my students on accomplishing what is often the hardest part of an exercise regimen—"getting here." Whether you find fulfillment in a class, taking the dog for a walk around the block, or walking/running up and down the stairs for fifteen minutes a day in your home or apartment building, do something that is accessible to you, energizes you, gets your endorphins flowing, and makes you feel good. A girlfriend of mine cranks up the music on her MP3 player, puts her headphones on, and dances around her living room for exercise when she can't get to the gym (her grade school kids are only slightly mortified when they witness this practice). "Find something you like to do and do it on a regular basis," says a veteran mom of two teenagers. Nike's "Just Do It" slogan has been successful for a reason. It is simple, it is empowering, and it doesn't tell you what to do or how to do it; it tells you just to take action and *do something* good for yourself. This "something" does not mean that you have to attend a spin class three times a week, or sign up for tennis league or running club. It relates to Woody Allen's message: *showing up* means taking care of yourself and your body. Here are some suggestions on how to show up for you:

◆ Show up on your yoga mat in your basement to practice for twenty minutes before your kids get up.
◆ Show up on your driveway or front steps to shovel snow after it falls (what a workout that is!).
◆ Show up in the front yard to throw the football around with your son (pretty soon he will say no because it won't be "cool" for him to be seen playing football with his mom).
◆ Show up in your family room to put on an exercise video, or even Wii Fit. Who knows, maybe your kids and your partner will join in the fun!
◆ Show up in your living room for a dance party that maybe only you attend.

It may take you a while to figure out what type of movement feels good to you, and how and when you will fit it in (before the kids get up, after they go to bed, or with them included or nearby). Your choice of activity may change—it's actually really good to switch things up periodically. But after a while, moving your body will become an integral, positive, and joyful component of your self-care solution. It will be harder for you to *not* do it than to listen to Nike (but with self-compassion in mind).

The benefits of exercise and good nutrition are countless, and some are more obvious than others. They are found in numerous research studies and revealed in almost every women's magazine. They include:

◆ Mood elevation
◆ Reduction or even elimination of depression and anxiety
◆ Better sleep
◆ Weight loss
◆ Increased sex drive

- Increased self-esteem
- Reduction of risk for disease and dis-ease

Moms are well aware that their bodies are meant to "move it or lose it," and that they are to be well nourished (how crazy are we about properly nourishing our children?). Without these two integral self-care components, your self-care solution will not be complete.

As much as we can try to control our health through making healthy choices about food and exercise, there is another essential component to physical self-care that sometimes can be underplayed or overlooked. While most moms would never neglect to take their baby in for his six-week or six-year checkup, many mothers are far less diligent about making yearly visits to the doctor themselves. The following list will (I hope) seem elementary to most, but there are too many stories of women ignoring certain signals in their bodies and not seeking medical care for something that could have been very manageable and treatable but, left untreated, turned into something very serious or, in some cases, deadly.

- Go to the doctor. Like clockwork. Every year. Do not skip a year because you are too busy with the kids and work. Getting your yearly physical is just as important as getting your children theirs. Be honest with your doctor about how you are feeling physically, mentally, and emotionally.
- Get regular mammograms when your doctor instructs you to. Do not skip a year because you are "fine." Do breast self-exams.
- See a dermatologist once a year. Have your body examined for irregular looking or growing "spots" or moles.
- Listen, *really listen*, to your body. If something doesn't feel right, do not ignore it. Get it checked out and let your doctor tell you that you are "fine."

- If you are in pain, your body is trying to tell you something. Be proactive about seeking help (physical therapy, chiropractic work, massage, acupuncture) for an aching back, neck or knee (or any other body part). A little knee pain can turn into a big knee surgery if you ignore the your body's signals and do nothing to take care of it. And it is hard to really feel happy when something hurts all the time.
- Go to the dentist every six months. Take care of your smile so you feel good about sharing it often.

And I would be remiss if I didn't add these life-and-death self-care tips:

- Wear your seat belt. Always.
- Don't text and drive. Really.
- Don't drink and drive. Just don't.

SELF-CARE LIVES FAR BENEATH THE SURFACE OF THE BODY

While I was fully recovered from my eating disorder by the time I became a mom, and although I have not fallen back into those extreme types of destructive patterns, the issues relating to perfectionism, self-acceptance, and self-compassion that led me to become anorexic at age seventeen are issues that I still deal with at forty-eight. Thankfully, I have been married to a man for twenty-two years who has been a constant support and sounding board for me in this area (his love for me, and for my changing body throughout four pregnancies and their aftermaths, has been unwavering). I also continue to spend time on my yoga mat, in meditation, and in talking to trusted friends and family members, all of which provide the continual and essential reminders that self-care is self-love, and self-love lives far beneath the surface of the physical body.

For me to stay centered and balanced, and to be the kind of person, mom, friend, and wife I want to be, I know that I need to do this work. Even if you have never suffered from an eating disorder, doing anything that involves connecting with yourself on a deeper level will most certainly allow for any food, exercise, or body image "battles" to become much less daunting. This shift will increase the probability that real, sustainable changes will occur, not only in this area of self-care but others as well. For many moms who struggle in this area of self-care, making lasting changes is much more complicated than just making a commitment to eat better and exercise more. A good portion of the moms I surveyed admitted that they repeatedly hit roadblocks in their self-care approach as it related to food and exercise. Oftentimes, focusing on the external factors alone (as in what food you are consuming and how much you are exercising) is not enough to bring about lasting and positive changes.

Mothers who are overweight sometimes jump on the yo-yo dieting and exercise train and never quite find their natural "sweet spot." They need to feel comfortable in their own bodies without feeling like they are punishing or depriving themselves through restrictive dieting or joyless, calorie-burning exercise, which is not very fun or sustainable. So, eventually, they just give up and stop trying. Other mothers may be able to maintain a "healthy" weight, but their external focus on food, exercise, and body image drives them to obsessive and sometimes destructive levels of exercising, extreme rigidity around food and compulsive calorie-counting, an unhealthy focus on body image, and an unhealthy determination to obtain and maintain washboard abs and "buns of steel." Both of these scenarios are counterproductive to any self-care plan, and neither of them is a healthy model for our children.

Goals related to food and exercise need not be attached to what the scale says, how many calories you are consuming a day, or whether or not you would be caught dead in a bikini. *The real goal for your self-care solution in this area needs to be focused on how you* feel—*your energy level, your mood, and your level of acceptance, love, and appreciation for your body.*

After many years of trial and error, I have come to a pretty decent understanding of what combinations of food and exercise work for my mind and body. I do not weigh myself, but I do know when my jeans are too tight. My understanding of how my body works and what it needs for me to thrive, physically and mentally, goes far beyond keeping my weight healthy and stable. I have developed an awareness of and respect for my body's signals, and I am intentional about listening to and honoring those signals. I knew, when I began to suffer from ongoing back and neck pain, that it was time to stop running. Now when I go for walks, either alone or with a friend, I feel good. I have learned that when I get "too busy" and don't practice yoga at least once or twice a week, I am way more stressed-out and irritable. When I don't sleep enough, or when I don't eat a well-balanced diet, I feel lethargic and am far less productive. I know that when I eat lots of sugary foods—which I love—I vacillate between feeling agitated and jittery and feeling exhausted (and yet I do still indulge from time to time). I learned that mixing yoga with weights and high-impact cardio in bare feet (yoga sculpt—a class I taught for four years) caused discs to bulge in my spine, and that I needed to choose another type of kinder, gentler yoga to teach and practice.

For many women, food and exercise addictions are often swept under the rug, and yet they can have hazardous effects on a mother's self-worth. Furthermore, a mother's negative patterns around food and body image are often unwittingly passed on to her children. Maternal concerns about body weight may be the third leading cause of body image problems in adolescents, according to a study by Harvard Medical School researchers.[8]

The most crucial component in finding peace in your relationships with food and movement is to listen to what your body tells you, and to be very honest with yourself about if, when, and how you use food or exercise as a numbing agent. This is often the biggest and most difficult obstacle for moms to overcome.

Once a woman's relationship with food and her body takes a

negative turn, it can become extremely difficult to break unhealthy thought and behavior patterns. As Wendy Mogel explains in her book *The Blessing of a Skinned Knee*, "Women in particular often harbor a deep, private love-hate relationship with food. Many distrust a substance they must rely on to stay alive but fear will lead them to lose control, overeat, and gain weight."[9]

Alcoholics need to abstain from the substance they use to numb themselves from stress or pain. But abstaining from food or movement is not the "solution" to food or exercise-related issues, because we need food and movement for survival. To truly find peace with food and our bodies, and to ensure that food becomes a positive element in our lives and the lives of our children, it is important to examine our practices around food, eating, and family meals. Mogel continues, "We are not to deny ourselves the joy of eating or to make an idol of food. There is a third possibility we must also avoid: consuming food without any thought at all, like beasts. Animals eat alone and on the run; they eat to survive, not to savor. They don't cook, arrange the food on the plate, or set a nice table."[10]

THE HEALTHY ROLE MODEL
FOR YOUR CHILDREN—YOU

It is essential for mothers to be honest about their relationship with food, not only because they need nourishment to keep themselves healthy so they can feel good and take care of their families, but also because mothers play a significant role in a child's attitude toward food and body image. The most powerful way to teach children healthy eating habits is through example. It is not enough simply to talk about nutrition and to force your children to eat good food, keeping the "bad" food from them. They will find the bad food soon enough, and undoubtedly they will turn to *you* for a real-life example of what a healthy relationship with food looks like. My mother battled with food and body image issues while I was growing up, and while I know that she was not aware of how closely I was watching her—and that she never intended to cause me any harm—this was a source of a great deal of confusion and fear for me. Now that I have my own children, I'm even more aware of how big an impact a mother can have on her kids, and that's part of why I'm so committed to being diligent about self-care. I want to do my best to ensure that I model the important lessons about nourishment and its relationship to self-love, self-respect, and self-acceptance that I want my children to absorb as they mature. Am I always able to be a great example to my children in this area? No, of course there are times when I am stressed or overwhelmed and therefore don't care for myself as well as I should. However, I have found that the key is to keep the communication open. Talk openly and honestly about food and exercise with your children. Teach them about nutrition so that they can gain a deep understanding of what their bodies and their minds need to grow and be healthy. And be careful about the way in which, and how frequently, you talk about your own, your kids', and other people's body size and shape. There is already an overemphasis on body image and physical appearance in society, so you can give your children a gift by teaching them about the importance of self-care and being a good person, instead of focusing too much on their physical appearance or the appearance of others.

If you are struggling to find your own balance in this area, your kids are another great reason for you to deal with any underlying issues that may be contributing to your food battles. If you can't seem to tackle them on your own, make sure to seek guidance, healing, or inspiration from a trusted friend, spiritual advisor, or therapist.

From my personal experience, my research, and my interviews with moms, it is clear to me that if a mother is willing to do the sometimes uncomfortable emotional work of asking herself the difficult questions—how she truly feels about herself and her body, what her relationship with food entails and how she formed this relationship, about how she copes with stress, whether or not she has a healthy support system and, if not, how she is going to create one—then and only then can she become deeply, internally connected with herself, her body, and her needs.

Starting from a place of self-awareness and self-acceptance allows you to more easily access and decipher the signals of your body and mind, and to understand what you truly need and don't need.

Instead of being blocked or controlled by all sorts of shoulds and shouldn'ts, goods and bads, the choice to fill yourself up with an adequate amount of nutrient-rich food and to approach exercise in a healthy, safe, enjoyable, and sustainable manner is a way to honor yourself every day. The mothers I surveyed who claimed to be the happiest and most balanced have always incorporated exercise and good nutrition into their motherhood self-care routines. They have connected the dots between making healthy choices, feeling good, and being a better, more energetic, happy, and present mom:

> *I take good care of myself by taking time to run, practice yoga and just be physical! A healthy mom is a happy mom!*
>
> —MOTHER OF FOUR CHILDREN,
> *ages eighteen, sixteen, fourteen, and twelve*

> *I've always taken good care of myself. If you don't model that, how will your kids know to do it? I think when kids see behavior (good and bad) they repeat it. For example: eating healthy food . . . trust me, they want to eat all the crap and you can't ban all crap, but again, they thank me today for teaching them to have healthy eating habits.*
>
> —MOTHER OF TWO CHILDREN,
> *ages twenty-two and twenty*

These moms do provide wonderful inspiration—but, yes, many moms feel that these practices are much easier said than done. Most moms do want to take care of themselves and provide good examples for their children, but the reality is that they won't be perfect at it all the time. Sticking with the same routine for twenty years is much more of the exception than the norm. Many of us can recall the several times we have vowed to start an exercise program, which we begin with a bang—and yet, by the end of the first week we are tired and sore, and we decide to take the next week off, and that week turns into a year. We promise that we will start making healthy meals for our family, but after work and kids' sports practices, everyone is so exhausted (especially Mom) that opting for the McDonald's drive-through sounds much easier than cooking the chicken broccoli stir-fry we had intended to make. We know how good chocolate tastes when we are stressed or lonely, or how we break out the Doritos when we are so angry with our spouse that we want to say all sorts of horrible things we know we will regret.

Once in a while there is no real harm in losing yourself in a jar of peanut butter (don't forget the chocolate chips) after a really tough week at work or with the kids, or stopping to pick up takeout for your family because you are too tired to cook, or occasionally taking some time off from your exercise routine. However, because moms are continually pushed and pulled in so many different directions, if the breaks go too long and you find yourself veering further and further off course, it becomes more and more challenging to move yourself back on track.

Prolonged periods of detaching your mind from your body pull you away from your core and your center, from what you instinctively know is right for you and for your family. And after a while, you almost become numb to the healthy signals and cues your body and mind give you. You stop being intentional about doing what you know and feel is good for you, and move into survival mode.

However, for most moms, it is possible to do more than just survive (although there will certainly be times when you truly are just happy to have made it through the day). In order to move from surviving to thriving, it is essential that you stay connected with your sense of self and keep your mind-body connection strong. Here are some very simple reminders to help you do this:

- Slow down (really, just try).
- Take deep, belly-expanding breaths (which will help you feel like you are able to slow down a bit).
- Ask for help when you need it.
- Say kind things to yourself like: "I am good enough," "I am doing the best I can," "I am worthy of good food and healthy movement, and eating good food and moving my body will help me feel good and stay healthy."
- Embrace the changes that occur in your body during pregnancy. Utilize the self-care principles regarding nourishment and movement outlined in this book, both during pregnancy and after.
- Be careful to recognize extreme thoughts and behaviors that can be unhealthy and destructive, like "I am going to eat everything in sight because I am pregnant," or "Now that I have had the baby, I am going to drastically restrict my intake so I lose the baby weight quickly," or "I am already fat and I don't have the time or energy to lose the weight, so why bother?"
- Be kind to yourself. Be kind to your body. Be patient with yourself and your body. Use moderation in your thoughts and actions.

Whether you are pregnant, going through menopause, or anywhere in between, know that it will not always be easy to find your equilibrium as hormones rage and metabolisms shift without warning. But staying connected to yourself and your body's signs and signals will help you stay grounded in your overall self-care solution, and specifically in the areas of nourishment and movement.

ESSENTIAL SELF-CARE TOOLS FOR MOVEMENT AND NOURISHMENT, INSIDE AND OUT

While it is helpful for most moms to be deliberate and methodical about food intake and exercise, the best-laid plans do go astray now and then. And that's okay. As a mother, you need to have a certain amount of flexibility—and the ability to find your way back to a healthy equilibrium if you decide to splurge on burgers, fries, and a milkshake with your kids, or if your Fitbit is flashing you nasty messages because you have not walked your usual ten thousand steps in several days. Always keep in mind that a healthy approach to food and exercise starts from within, where self-respect, self-love, and, ultimately, your commitment to self-care resides.

THE BASICS

If you are looking to make changes or enhancements to your approach to your physical self-care, it is essential for you to step back and do an honest self-assessment in your approach to food, exercise, sleep, and your feelings about your body. Questions to ask yourself include:

- ◆ Do you like your body? Why or why not?
- ◆ If you do not like your body, how often do you think about your dissatisfaction with it? Do you share these feelings with your partner/with your children?
- ◆ Do your feelings about your body affect your sex life? Do you not want to be touched? Do you feel unattractive?
- ◆ Are you at a healthy weight (within five to ten pounds of the "appropriate" weight for your height/build)? You can check with your doctor if you are not sure.
- ◆ Do you want to lose (or gain) a few (or many) pounds? Why or why not?
- ◆ How often do you think about food? When you are hungry? Most of the day? How often do you try to avoid thinking about food?
- ◆ Do you eat when you are hungry and stop when you are full?
- ◆ Do you plan your meals? For yourself and for your family?

- How do you feel about exercise? Are there activities
  that you like to do that involve movement?
  What are they?
- Do you binge-eat and/or binge-exercise?
- Do you diet?
- How many hours of sleep per night do you need
  to feel alert and rested the next day?
- How many hours do you actually sleep each night?

In order to create healthy and constructive pathways around
food, exercise, and sleep, it is essential to formulate a realistic
regimen that is flexible, positive, affirming, and steady. Here are
some simple yet essential tools for developing a manageable,
grounded, and sustainable approach to food and exercise:

- Focus less on "diet," and more on steadily filling
  up your body with wholesome, nutrient-rich food
  and lots of water.
- Become educated about what you are putting into
  your body. Learn about nutrition, about
  whole foods, about processed foods. Watch the
  documentaries Food Inc., Forks Over Knives,
  and Super Size Me. Read It Starts With Food, by
  Dallas and Melissa Hartwig, and explore healthy
  food websites that include a plethora of great
  recipes, like Blue Zones, Deliciously Ella, and
  Nourished Kitchen.
- When exercising, think less about "calorie burning,"
  and more about the importance of daily movement
  for your mind and body.
- Listen to your body during and after exercise.
  Be kind to yourself even if you enjoy the feeling of
  high-intensity, rigorous workouts. Remember that
  the "no pain, no gain" mantra can lead to serious
  injury. Understand the difference between
  discomfort, which is usually okay to push through,

and pain, which most often is a signal to back off.

◆ Listen to your body's food-related signals, both when hungry and when satiated, and honor those signals.

◆ Notice how your emotional state is connected to when and how you eat. Do you eat more when you are bored, tired, upset? Or do you skip meals when you are stressed? Do you eat over the kitchen sink, in the car, or when you are alone? Late at night?

◆ Make a concerted effort to sit down and eat meals, especially an evening meal with your family.

◆ When you wake up in the morning, take a moment to find gratitude—gratitude that your body is healthy and will do the majority of what you ask it to do, and gratitude that you have the ability to make good choices about what foods you will put in your body.

◆ Start the day with a good, healthy breakfast. This one is so important, and yet so often gets skipped by moms who, ironically, are hell-bent on making sure their kids get something nutritious in their bodies before they leave for school or day care (because they do know how important it is). As John L. Ivy, an emeritus professor of health education at the University of Texas at Austin, writes, "Breakfast immediately raises the energy level of the body, increasing vigor and vitality. It reduces blood cortisol levels and helps control appetite, which over the long-term, can significant impact body composition. Breakfast also increases cognitive function and the ability to concentrate."[11]

◆ Before you eat something, take a moment to appreciate the food, whether it is by saying a prayer or just by acknowledging that food is something to be appreciated and not taken for granted.

Connect with gratitude before and after you exercise—gratitude for the movement of your body, and gratitude that you made a choice to do something good for yourself.

MOVEMENT
Do you feel that you incorporate enough body movement into your day? If not, what gets in your way? How could you incorporate ten minutes of sustained movement into your life every day? Fifteen minutes?

List ten specific activities that you could commit to doing four to five days a week that involve moving your body for at least twenty minutes. Suggestions:

◆ Walk up and down the stairs in your home, apartment building, or office.
◆ Choose the stairway over the elevator or escalator.
◆ Take your dog for a walk.
◆ Walk at the mall.
◆ Play soccer with your child.
◆ Join a tennis league.
◆ Take classes at a local health club or recreation center.
◆ Park in the spot furthest from the entrance whenever you go to work, Target, or the grocery store or doctor's office, and walk that extra minute or two from car to building and back.
◆ Ride your bike.
◆ Shovel snow.

List ten activities that you have never tried, or have not done in a long time, that you would be willing to give the old college try (even just once). Suggestions:

◆ Cross-country skiing
◆ Snowshoeing
◆ Ice skating
◆ Roller skating

- Jumping rope
- Square dancing
- Line dancing
- Zumba
- Swimming (really, when was the last time you got in the water and really swam, not just splashed around with your kids?)
- Softball
- Frisbee

Other creative suggestions:

- When you are watching your kids play sports, instead of spending that entire hour or two sitting on the bleachers, wear your sneakers and walk around the soccer, football, or baseball field while you watch your little guy or girl. (It's little trickier for basketball and hockey, but walking up and down the bleacher stairs a few times at halftime instead of getting a hot dog may be just what you really need. Who cares what the other parents say? Maybe they will join you.)
- When you are at home with the kids, do as much walking around your house or apartment as you can: pick up and deliver laundry to the kids' rooms with a smile, knowing you are getting more steps in; throw in a few lunges as you walk down the hall; take yourself back to fifth grade gym class and take a stab at a few rounds of push-ups, sit-ups, or jumping jacks, and maybe throw in a few burpees just for fun.
- Invest in exercise, yoga, or meditation CDs and DVDs (and then do the hardest part: open them and try them out).
- For working moms: if you typically sit at a desk all day, make sure to check your posture regularly, stand up periodically, and take a lap or two around

the office to get your blood flowing to your mind and muscles as often as you can. A 2013 study by scientists from Maastricht University in the Netherlands recommends five minutes of standing for every thirty minutes of sitting.[12] Keep handheld weights nearby and ignore stares from coworkers as you stand and do a few sets of curls throughout the workday. Take a walk during part of your lunch break, or take a brisk walk around the block at the end of your workday, to clear your mind and to give yourself some renewed energy before you hop in the car and pick up the kids from day care or head home.

NOURISHMENT

Envision what you want your food and exercise plan to look like. Set small goals. Suggestions:

◆ Drink more water.
◆ Eat more vegetables.
◆ Notice your sugar intake—maybe cut out one sugary item (like soda) that you consume regularly.
◆ Notice when and how you eat—in the car, standing in the kitchen, late at night, when you are bored, sad, or tired.
◆ Connect with your body's signals of hunger and satiety.

Create healthy patterns around food for yourself and for your family. Describe your relationship with food and what kind of role food plays in your life and in your family's life. How could you add more joy and meaning into nourishing yourself and nourishing your family? Suggestions:

◆ Make sure that there is joy in your kitchen: play music; engage your kids in meal planning, preparation, and clean-up.
◆ Do your best to sit down as a family and eat together as

often as possible. Our family does our very best to have Friday night Shabbat dinners together. If everyone in your family is on a different schedule and you all tend to eat on the run, try to schedule at least one family meal together during the week; maybe it's Saturday brunch (before Joey's soccer game) or Sunday dinner.

◆ If you notice that you have become something of a short order cook and often find yourself standing at the kitchen sink eating food off your kids' plates instead of sitting down with your family and enjoying a meal together, try to at least sit down with them for a few minutes, and engage them in conversation.

◆ Be intentional about preparing healthy meals for yourself and your family (especially on hectic nights).

◆ Develop meal plans, cook in advance, and freeze meals that can easily be heated and served.

◆ If you feel frustrated about your diet or your family's diet, take an honest look at what gets in the way of your making positive changes, like time constraints, exhaustion, and picky eaters (e.g., "Okay, you can have mac and cheese for the fourth night in a row because I am too tired to battle with you over eating a protein and a vegetable").

◆ What small but positive changes could you make?

◆ Always remember that it is essential to nourish yourself and your family with good, healthy food. Yes, doing so takes more effort and attention, and sometimes money. However, keep in mind that while fresh fruits and vegetables are more expensive than packaged and processed foods, they are much cheaper than medical expenses related to poor health and obesity.

Nourishing and moving your body are essential components of self-care and are directly linked to self-love, self-respect, and self-compassion. Physically caring for yourself sends an ongoing message to you and those around you, especially your children, that you value your health and that it is important that they value theirs. It is important that you are *mindful* (not obsessive) about exercise and nutrition—not because you need to be concerned about what you look like in a bikini, but because your health is important for you and for your family, and because physically feeling good allows you to have the energy and stamina to manage all of your responsibilities as a woman and as a mother.

CHAPTER 4:

Self-Care Solution #2— Embrace Sleep and Rest

Because of the prevalence of statements like "I'll sleep when I'm dead" or "Sleep is for the weak," moms can sometimes feel that sleep is just a luxury, a waste of time, and needs to be placed at the very end of their never-ending list of priorities. I see moms drop their eyes in shame when they *whisper* an *admission* that they took a nap during the day. Well, sleep experts will tell you that this shame must be left out on the curb with the rest of the garbage. Taking care of your body and mind by providing it with adequate rest is a hugely important aspect of self-care.

IN THE BEGINNING

Although many moms feel as if they "should" be doing something much more productive than sleeping when their baby sleeps, researchers beg to differ. The negative effects of sleep deprivation are real and can cause lasting damage. According to a 2013 article by Seth Maxon on the website of *The Atlantic*, "Losing sleep can cause hallucinations, psychosis, and long-term memory impairment. Some studies have linked sleep deprivation to chronic conditions like hypertension, diabetes, and bipolar disorder."

The National Heart, Lung, and Blood Institute recommends seven to eight hours of sleep per night. Getting less sleep than this can cause weight gain and decreased attention span and cognitive ability—none of which sounds attractive to anyone, let alone new moms. So it is imperative for new moms to enter their motherhood journey with an understanding of the importance of sleep. Mothers concur that the infant stage (which lasts only for about six months) is by far the most challenging from a sleep perspective, but once someone becomes a mother, she never sleeps quite the same as she used to. Talk to any mother of a teenager (especially one who is driving) and she will most likely reveal that she now sleeps with one eye open.

It is impossible for moms to be able to get the exact number of sleep hours needed every night (especially in the beginning), so do not be hard on yourself if it takes you a while to try different ways of grabbing sleep during your child's newborn stage. But in the spirit of self-care, and with your desire to be a healthy, balanced, present, and engaged mom, make sure you commit yourself to caring for yourself by getting as much sleep as you can. Here are a few tips for new moms on how to do that:

- Sleep when your baby sleeps (day and night).
- Be consistent with your baby's bedtime as soon as you can.
- Unplug: turn off your cell phone, computer, and tablet when the baby is sleeping so you are not tempted to be sucked into the time warp of social media.
- Ask for help! Have your partner do some of the feedings (pump milk if you are breastfeeding). Ask grandma to take the baby overnight and catch up on some much needed sleep.
- Ask a friend or neighbor to come over during the day so you can take a nap. Who doesn't want to hold a newborn for a few hours?
- If your budget allows, hire a babysitter or someone to come in every so often and help with housework. And use this time to rest.
- If any of your friends or family members offer to

bring meals for you and your family when you come home from the hospital, say yes! This will allow you to spend less with meal preparation and more time sleeping or resting.

◆ Let go—*really* let go—of many of your shoulds that pull you away from sleep: cleaning your house, returning e-mail and phone calls, writing thank-you notes for baby gifts. People understand that the most important thing you need right now is to take care of yourself and your baby (and if they don't understand this, they aren't your real friends).

As a new mother, transitioning into one of the most important and most selfless roles you will ever have, the sooner you get in the habit of prioritizing your needs, the easier it will be to stay committed to doing so for the long haul. And adequate sleep is a hugely important part of your self-care solution. You need sustained energy and an alert mind to properly take care of your baby, and being well rested (and well nourished) will help you be able to do that the way you want to.

Authors Dean Raffelock, Robert Rountree, Virginia Hopkins, and Melissa Block reveal the importance of sleep for new moms in their book, *A Natural Guide to Pregnancy and Postpartum Health*: "In our experience, the mothers who stay particularly healthy postpartum are the ones who allow themselves to sleep as much as they feel necessary. Most say that they took two- to three-hour naps every day for the first six months of their babies' lives. They didn't jump up to clean house or cook or pay bills when baby fell asleep. When their babies slept, they slept."[13]

As most mothers quickly come to find out, as wonderful as it is to care for and nurture your new baby, the sleep deprivation can be overwhelmingly difficult. One mom of two young children described the infancy stage as "sort of like being in a torture facility. The sleepless nights can be almost unbearable at times. It becomes really hard to function." I can certainly relate to that feeling.

My second son was severely colicky. If he wasn't sleeping (and he wasn't, most of the time), he cried a bloodcurdling, fingernails-on-the-chalkboard shriek that sounded like he was writhing in pain, even though my pediatrician assured me he wasn't. There were countless sleepless nights when I buckled him into his car seat and drove around and around the neighborhood to try to lull him to sleep. The short periods of time that he would sleep during the day, I didn't sleep. In fact, I *couldn't* sleep—there were too many other things like laundry and dishes that I thought were more important than my sleep.

One day, I was taking a two-minute shower as my son was buckled into his car seat, positioned outside the shower door, and per usual, he was screaming his brains out. I suddenly felt a stabbing pain in my lower belly. I dropped to my knees and crawled my way out of the shower, grabbing the phone just as I doubled over and fell to the floor. I called my husband and he rushed home, not knowing whom to console first—our son, whose cries had not let up, or me. I thought for sure I was hemorrhaging and that I would most certainly bleed to death right there on the bathroom floor. But there was no blood. My husband whisked me and our crying son to my OB's office. After a few tests, my doctor told us that I checked out okay, and that if it happened again and there was any bleeding, to call right away. The pain did subside, but for the next several months I suffered from regular bouts of severe abdominal pain (and yet I did not call the doctor).

I was afraid to eat because I thought maybe I had developed a food sensitivity, and if I had, I was unsure of which foods would ignite the stomach spasms. The lack of nourishment (and sleep) made me agitated, fearful, and stressed, which all aggravated my stomach even more. There were many nights when my colicky son and I were both up crying inconsolably. At my husband's insistence, I finally consulted a GI doctor, and through the process of elimination, and undergoing further tests for ulcers, Crohn's disease, and colitis, I was finally diagnosed with irritable bowel syndrome. I learned that IBS often affects women in their early thirties, is often brought on by stress, and is aggravated by sleep deprivation and continual stress.

In retrospect, I know that I should have slept. My current self-care prescription would have told me to sleep, or at least rest when I could. But at the time, I didn't believe that. (Note to sleep deprived new mothers: sleep trumps laundry—always. And if you can't actually *sleep*, do not fret—just rest. Even closing your eyes for a few minutes on the couch is beneficial.)

◆ ◆ ◆

The trickiest part about self-care for moms is that there is so much about motherhood that we can't prepare for or control. I couldn't control that my son had colic and I certainly wasn't prepared for it. And this scared me to the core and also made me feel like I was failing him. I, like many of the women quoted in this book, found myself surrendering to his condition, thinking, *I can't take care of myself. I have to try to console him. And I can't sleep when he sleeps because I have to keep the house clean. My husband will be disappointed if the house is a mess when he gets home.*

This is the point when a mom's self-care voice needs to drown out the "shoulds" and the "can'ts." I fully needed to believe that taking care of my health was more important than the laundry being folded or the crumbs wiped off the kitchen counter. I also needed to replace the shame and guilt of not being able to console my crying baby with the concept that his colic was not my fault, and that I *could* put him down in a safe place when I needed to take a break from his crying and rest. I also needed to ask for help, which I finally did. We ended up hiring an amazing babysitter who would come in a few times a week and basically just be another set of arms for my crying son. But I still did not rest like I should. And my stomach problems continued for several years, long after the colic had subsided. In fact, it wasn't until I started doing yoga that they finally resolved.

My lack of sleep caused me to get sick. I did not listen closely enough to the signals my body was giving me. My story exemplifies the importance of finding ways to get adequate rest even during more stressful times. I know that during these difficult months I was exhausted, and did not give my baby or my three-year-old the kind of time and attention that I wanted to. I was not able to be the kind of mom I wanted to be because I did not take proper care of myself. As difficult as this lesson was, I am grateful that I learned about the importance of sleep relatively early on in my parenting journey. I was much more mindful about getting a decent amount of sleep when my next two children were babies, and I had a much more positive experience during their infant stages.

LATER ON

Once children begin sleeping through the night, a mom's sleep cycle usually returns to normal and she begins to feel human again. But sleep challenges often continue. Sickness, night terrors, or just wanting to be close to Mom and Dad can cause kids to find their way into parents' beds in the middle of the night. I will not engage in the debate about a family bed, but let's just say that my kids learned pretty early on that I am a light sleeper and that inadequate sleep absolutely does not work for me. So if they ever needed middle-of-the-night assistance or comforting, they usually woke my husband (and still do occasionally).

As for the wake-before-dawn stage that many kids go through, especially when they get into their big beds and can get out when they want to: as soon as the kids knew their numbers, I put digital clocks in their rooms. I told them that when they woke up in the morning, if the first number was anything less than a six (or a seven on the weekends), they could play quietly in their room until they saw the appropriate number. This worked like a charm! Teaching kids about the importance of sleep for themselves, and the importance of respecting mom's need for sleep, is an important part of your self-care solution. Kids need to understand that it is not okay to wake Mommy any time they feel like it, and that Mommy needs her sleep so she can be happy and fun to be with, not crabby and too tired to play with her children.

The teenage years will add new twists to the sleep challenge. Teens will stay up very late doing homework, chatting with their friends, perusing Facebook, watching shows, and checking fantasy football scores. Most cities and/or states have mandated curfews. In Hennepin County, Minnesota, it is eleven p.m. during the week and twelve a.m. on weekends, although many parents choose their own curfews that work for their families. It is an interesting transition when you find yourself going to bed before your child. But you need to take care of yourself, and you need to remind your teen to do so as well. Many teens think that they can function on far less sleep than they actually need. Although many teens will challenge you on this, six hours of sleep is not enough for a teenage brain to recharge itself. In fact, according to the National Sleep Foundation, teens need about eight to ten hours of sleep each night in order to function well.[14] And research show that only 15 percent of our teens are actually getting that.[15] Just as moms need to be proactive and intentional about getting adequate sleep, it is crucial to emphasize the importance of sleep to our children and to make sure they understand that sleep deprivation can have serious consequences. According to *The Atlantic*, "Chronic sleep loss contributes to higher rates of depression, suicidal ideation, and obesity. Long-term deprivation has also been shown to be a factor in lower test scores, decreased attention span, tardiness, concentration, and overall academic achievement."[16]

Establishing firm bedtimes for your kids for as long as you can truly enforce them, as well as committing to a healthy bedtime for yourself, are important strategies in making the sure the whole family is well rested. For me, my biggest challenge is unplugging. I stay up too late writing, returning e-mails, checking Facebook, and reading on my Kindle, which, according to new research, is the worst thing I can be doing before trying to fall asleep. In 2012, researchers at Rensselaer Polytechnic Institute found that exposure to light from computer tablets lowered levels of the hormone melatonin, which regulates our internal clock and helps us get a good night's rest.[17]

In other words, I would be much better off taking a hot bath and going straight to bed. Whatever your bedtime ritual is, make sure that it includes some kind of a wind-down that preferably does not involve a screen. Remember that books are still available in both hardcover and paperback.

The same underlying message—"I am worth it"—that propels you to take care of yourself by exercising and nourishing your body with good food and lots of water, also needs to move you to get adequate rest. Being intentional about getting your seven hours of sleep a night will allow you to wake up most mornings feeling rested and energized. Starting the day from this position of strength enables you to have more energy to exercise, make good decisions about your food intake, and take care of your family with enthusiasm and joy.

SLEEP TIPS FOR MOMS OF NEWBORNS
- Sleep when the baby sleeps. Really, it is that simple.
- When you can't fall asleep, just rest.
- Ask for help.

FOR MOMS OF OLDER CHILDREN
- Be diligent about bedtime, for your children and for yourself.
- Take a hot bath or read a book to relax before going to sleep.
- Avoid electronic gadgets before bed.

FOR MOMS OF TEENS
- Model healthy habits around sleep, and don't be afraid to go to sleep before your teens do.
- Encourage teens to get adequate rest and discuss its importance. Continue to challenge their assertion that they are "fine" going to bed at one a.m. and getting up at six thirty.
- Enforce a curfew that works for your family (so you don't have to be up until two a.m. waiting for your teens).

FOR ALL MOMS

- ◆ How many hours of sleep do you need a night to feel rested?
- ◆ How many hours do you actually sleep a night?
- ◆ If you are falling short on sleep hours, what is stopping you from getting adequate rest?
- ◆ Can you commit to trying to employ one or two of the above-mentioned tactics to increase your amount of sleep, even by a half hour a night?

CHAPTER 5:

Self-Care Solution #3— Cultivate Happiness and Joy

"We must make room for joy whenever it decides to show its mischievous face. And we must do this consistently, indefinitely."

—*Thelma Adams*

Taking care of your physical body through healthy nourishment, movement, and adequate sleep is an essential piece of your self-care solution that can be measured and monitored. These practices provide you with a solid foundation to be the best you can be for you and your family. But in order to be fully alive and engaged in your life, you must also continually tap into the power and importance of happiness, joy, and gratitude. *Crazy Sexy Cancer* author Kris Carr reiterates this message in her interview with mindbodygreen.com, "It's important to remember that everything is connected between the mind and the body. You can eat all that organic food and do all that yoga but if you're angry or stressed, much of the goodness goes to waste."

Feeding yourself emotionally, mentally, and spiritually is a critical component of your self-care prescription—not to mention the best gift you can give the people you love and care about. As one mother of two children, ages nineteen and seventeen, explained, "Ultimately, a mother's happiness certainly impacts the climate of her home and the feelings that she emits to her children and partner. A happy mom is key to a happy home!"

As mothers know, caring for children can feel all-consuming, draining, exhausting, and downright terrifying, and can also make it difficult for us to continually remind ourselves that we are women, separate from our children, and that we are worthy of feeling happiness, contentment, and inner peace. Although it is virtually impossible for anyone to feel those emotions all the time, moms need to keep their pulse on their innermost passions, hopes, and dreams, and try to live them out in some measure as often as they can, *while* their children are living in the house. Although they may have to do some shifting of priorities and put some of their bucket-list items on the back burner for a while, mothers need not feel like they must put their own happiness and fulfillment on hold entirely when parenting their children. In other words, *don't let your kids be the only thing you care deeply about or the only aspect of your life that brings you joy.*

In fact, now is as good a time as any to take a few moments to do a happiness check-in by asking yourself some important questions:

- How do you define happiness? What does happiness look and feel like to you?
- Are you happy? With yourself? With your relationship with your partner? Your friends? Your children?
- If not, how could you be happier?
- Do you know what makes you happy?
- When was the last time you felt pure joy?
- When was the last time you laughed until your stomach hurt? Or even just laughed?

If you answered "I don't know," "no," or "I can't remember" to more than a few of these questions, it is probably time to make some changes in an effort to cultivate more happiness within yourself and within your life. But why, you might ask, is it so important for you to be happy?

I will never forget a saying that one of my counselors, Stu, shared with me at the age of seventeen when I was locked up in an adolescent psych ward for my eating disorder. (There were no specific eating disorder treatment facilities in the early eighties—or at least there were none in Minnesota). I was complaining about something to him; maybe it was about my family, my school, or myself. But basically, I was telling him I was unhappy. And he said to me, "Don't you know the saying, 'Life sucks and then you die'?"

No, I didn't—and I did not like the sound of it. Maybe he was being flippant. Maybe he wanted me to stop complaining and "get over myself." Maybe he was having a bad day (except that I vaguely remember a plaque with those words on it sitting on his desk). Needless to say, considering the weak and depressed state I was in when I heard it, that phrase haunted me for years—I mean, it *really* haunted me. I believed that maybe it was true, and that depressed me even more. Thankfully (and no thanks to him), throughout my recovery, as I began to open myself up to and experience more joy in my life, I came to learn not only that Stu was one hundred percent wrong in sharing that statement with a depressed and anxious anorexic patient, but that it could not be further from the truth. I am so happy to be able to report now, thirty years later, as a healthy, thriving mother of four, that life definitely does *not* suck, nor should that be the expectation! (For Stu's sake, and for that of the patients he subsequently worked with, I hope he also changed his tune.)

Just ask Gretchen Rubin, researcher and author of *The Happiness Project*, who has passionately poured herself into helping people understand the essential nature of happiness and joy. Had I known Rubin as she is today when I was seventeen, I am certain she would have encouraged me to remain hopeful and to continue to find the joy in life. And she would have told me what she tells her readers, quoting Aristotle: "'Happiness is the meaning and purpose of life, the whole aim and end of human existence.'"[18]

As is the case for most mothers, there have been times when my heart has been elevated to euphoric levels of happiness, and times when I've felt such despair (especially when a child experiences pain or suffering) that I've dropped to my knees begging for mercy. Despite the fact that I yearned to become a mother (four times over), and that motherhood has taken my existence and purpose in life to a level that I did not even know was possible, I have sometimes wanted to run away and hide when hearing one of my children utter the word "Mom." I have found myself wondering, from a more universal perspective, how having children affects a woman's overall happiness.

I was relieved to learn that I was not the only one pondering this question. Some studies show that "parenting is associated with decreased well-being,"[19] while others indicate that people with children are happier than those without them. As a mother of four, I prefer to ascribe to the latter idea, although I do appreciate the fact that these studies validate the reality of how draining motherhood can be.

The overall results of the studies support the conclusion that people (whether married or not) with children are happier, and experience more positive emotions and a deeper sense of meaning in their lives, than people who do not have children. (Interestingly enough, dads reported having even greater satisfaction than moms. Go figure!)

In an article in *Psychology Today*, the clinical psychologist and positive psychology expert Todd B. Kashdan writes:

> *Don't get me wrong, just as the headlines like to shout, parenting is hard and there are moments when it sucks. And once in a while, you might have that itchy feeling concerning the lost self: the past version of you, prior to parenthood, when you were responsible for no one else, when you could stay out all night with friends, dance on car hoods and wake up naked in a thorn bush with a smile of contentment.*
>
> *But you have to ask yourself a few things. What*

is so important in your life that you would die for it? What is so poignant that your eyes well up from joy? When you have an amazing moment with your children, don't let it go. Return to it when you're alone and recall that moment for 10 seconds. For 10 seconds, sit with it, close your eyes and savor it. Let it sink in. Because for many of us, these moments are the building blocks of the most meaningful life we will ever get.

So very, very true! So while it is important for moms to be mindful about holding on to their sense of self and to continue to foster happiness within themselves and with other relationships in their lives, it is also important to realize that embracing the joy, meaning, and sense of purpose found in motherhood as often as you can will boost your level of happiness.

◆ ◆ ◆

Step into any yoga class, and you most likely will be instructed to "stay present and focused on your mat." That advice can be directly applied to mothering. In yoga, you are moving through poses that can be very difficult and which can challenge you until you feel like you just can't move another muscle; the key is to stay focused on your breath, allow yourself to feel your power within, and continue to breathe. If you succeed in that, whether you back off from the pose or push through it, you realize that there is beauty in the dance that is happening on your mat—even if you find yourself resting in child's pose, merely focusing on the incredible sound and strength of your own breath. In motherhood, it is essential to allow yourself to breathe through the stress, aggravation, and heartache that you will inevitably face, and savor the true and incredible meaning of this role. By cherishing as many moments as you can along the way, you will be able to connect more deeply with the beautiful dance of motherhood and continually return to the meaningful building blocks that Kashdan describes.

To continually infuse your role as a mother with happiness and fulfillment, it is essential to be mindful and purposeful about your pursuit of happiness and fulfillment (which often go hand in hand):

- Seek out the joy in motherhood. Write down ten things that you love about being a mother to your children. Take time to step back and notice how amazing, wonderful, and sometimes magical this role is, and what an incredible influence you can have on your child's life. Allow yourself to feel joy about the big things and the smallest of things. For example, appreciate how you can literally wipe away little ones' pain with a kiss and a Band-Aid, and how you can share both your difficult and hilarious experiences with teens so they understand that although they will experience tough times, laughter and joy are always right around the corner.
- Laugh. A lot. Making sure there is humor and laughter in your home is an incredible way to provide much-needed levity for both you and your children. As Paul McGhee, Ph.D., writes, "Your sense of humor is one of the most powerful tools you have to make certain that your daily mood and emotional state support good health."
  - *Notice the number of times you laugh in one day. Strive to increase that number. There is no such thing as too much laughter (unless it is at the expense of others).*
  - *Notice what makes you laugh, as well as the people who make you laugh and bring you joy. Spend more with these people and in doing the things that make you laugh. (Watching Saturday Night Live reruns, Kristin Wiig's skits in particular, is a surefire way to send my daughters and me into fits of laughter. For many years, my husband would tell Jewish jokes to start our Friday night Shabbat dinners, attempting to end the week and begin the weekend with levity and laughter.)*
- List ten things about each of your children that make you smile. Share this list with your children and keep it handy for those times when you need a reminder.

- Write down what it feels like to love your child unconditionally.
- Write down what it feels like to be loved by your child.
- List ten activities that you do alone, with friends, with your partner, and with your children that you would describe as fun, and that bring you joy. Be intentional about weaving these activities into your life as often as you can.
- Dare to dream! Have you always wanted to go hang gliding? Write a book? Take up guitar? Pottery? Be open to trying new things that make you smile when you think about doing them.
- Tap into your creativity. Doodle, draw, paint, decorate, write, scrapbook, sing, play an instrument—anything that allows you to express yourself freely and ignite joy from within.

And take this wonderful advice from journalist and novelist Thelma Adams: "When I was a kid I loved to ride roller coasters—Disneyland's Matterhorn, Coney Island's rickety Cyclone. The slow ascent, the shivery pause at the top, the exhilarating drop: fun! How do we recapture that? By living in the moment—by being ready. Fun isn't an activity; it's the result of our willingness to be open. Fun is about spontaneity. It finds us when it wants to, and our job is to be ready."[20]

As part of my research, I asked mothers to take a moment to stop and reflect on motherhood and their level of happiness and contentment. Some mothers readily tapped into the joy and fulfillment (mixed in with some extra worry that goes with the territory) that they have experienced in becoming and being a mother, while other mothers revealed that they understand how self-care is directly tied into happiness:

I worry infinitely more, cherish every moment wholeheartedly, feel so important and valuable in a

truly meaningful, irreplaceable way, my heart has
opened wider than ever imaginable.

—MOTHER OF TWO CHILDREN, *ages eight and six*

I am content. I haven't been happy for a while. I feel
lost in my kids' world and cannot find my way back to
my own. I need to do some things for me to remember
who I used to be and who I want to be.

—MOTHER OF TWO CHILDREN,
ages three and one

I am attempting to be happy, but it is a slow process.
Being young, and now single with three kids under age
four is tough, but very rewarding. Sometimes I fear
that I need them too much, especially my 3 1/2 year old.
I am starting to realize that I need to develop a sense of
myself if I am going to be a good parent for them.

—MOTHER OF THREE CHILDREN,
ages three and one (twins)

I'm still working on how to be balanced, whole and
happy myself. I really think you have to nurture your
mind, body, and spirit.

—MOTHER OF TWO CHILDREN, *ages eleven and eight*

Other mothers revealed that, since becoming mothers, they felt
that seeking happiness for themselves was not their primary focus
anymore, and that taking care of their child (or children) and
their other responsibilities trumped all. As one mother reported:

I have moments of happiness and contentment, but
honestly I don't have enough time in the day to worry
about my feelings. I do what needs to be done and move
on to the next thing on the list.

—MOTHER OF THREE CHILDREN,
ages ten, eight, and five

Some moms claimed that they would be happier if their relationship with their partner were better, if they were in a more secure financial position, and if their kids were on track or not in crisis.

> *I do think I would be happier if I had time for me, if I felt like someone was as much invested in my well-being as I am in taking care of everyone else. It isn't so much happiness that I seek, but rather not feeling so alone.*
>
> —MOTHER OF THREE CHILDREN,
> ages ten, eight, and five

> *I am happiest when my husband and I are in sync; my kids are managing school and fun; my work is fulfilling (not too much work, not too little); my family and friends are available and not in crisis; and there is time left for fun and leisure. Seems easy enough but sometimes if just one of those is turbulent, it can affect my mood. In those situations, I try to reset my expectations from super happy to simply hopeful.*
>
> —MOTHER OF TWO CHILDREN,
> ages twenty-two and eighteen

Many moms expanded on the issue of how external forces (especially children) affected their levels of happiness, concurring with the statement "you are only as happy as your saddest child." Whether this rings true for you or not, most mothers agree that while moms usually do everything in their power to try to create an environment in which their children feel safe, loved, nurtured, and ultimately happy, it is very painful to learn that ultimately mothers cannot control the happiness of their children. There are so many other variables that children encounter in their lives, including dealing with their own chemistry, which mothers cannot control. But while mothers cannot control their children's happiness, they can certainly encourage it. "One of the best ways to make yourself happy is to make other people happy. One of the best ways to make other people happy is to be happy yourself," says Rubin.[21]

Moms need to place as much value on their mental and emotional well-being as they do on their physical. And while some people are hardwired to be more joyous or grumpier than others, Rubin reveals that "people have an inborn disposition that's set within a certain range, but they can boost themselves to the top of their happiness range or push themselves down to the bottom of their happiness range by their actions."[22] For me, I have found through my research, interviews, surveys, and forty-eight years of life experience—almost half of them as a mother—that staying deeply connected with myself and those around me is the most powerful way for me to feel happy as a human being, a partner, and a mother.

I find happiness in spending time alone reading, writing, or practicing yoga; I find happiness in spending time with my husband, whether it is taking a walk or taking a trip. I find happiness in spending time with good friends, and in being with my children, whether we are playing, watching a movie, or even doing homework. I find happiness in studying Judaism and in volunteering in the community. Some mothers I surveyed revealed that they find happiness in very simple pleasures like getting a haircut, "drinking Tim Hortons coffee," taking a ballet or a yoga class, going kayaking or hiking, gardening, painting, cooking, listening to music, dancing, going for a walk, quilting, painting their nails, reading, spending time with friends or partners, or watching movies or their favorite TV show. Other mothers revealed more elaborate ways in which they fill up their "happiness cup." Most importantly, what all of these mothers have in common is that they have identified what makes them happy and are committed to making their happiness-boosting activities a priority.

I would never tell my husband this, but I love to shovel snow. I even like to use the snowblower. There is something about being outside by myself, in the brisk

*cold, smelling the fresh air and getting some exercise
that invigorates me and makes me happy. But really,
don't tell my husband.*

—MOTHER OF TWO CHILDREN,
ages nine and seven

*I like to work out and that helps me recharge. I also
like talking with friends or just going on walks in the
neighborhood to see who's outside for an impromptu play
date. I participate in a book club, a MOPS [Mothers of
Preschoolers] group, and I take positions that force me to
use my brain—board chair of my son's pre-school, on the
local hockey rink board, group leader at MOPS.*

—MOTHER OF TWO CHILDREN,
ages five and two, and pregnant with a third

*I go away with girlfriends three weekends a year. When
I come back, I am happy, energized and refreshed. I
am a much better mother and am better able to handle
doing the mundane tasks that all mothers have to do.*

—MOTHER OF THREE CHILDREN
ages sixteen, fourteen, and eight

*I go out with girlfriends who make me laugh. I find
laughter to be my number one tonic! I also carve out
quiet time for reading and drawing. I enjoy opening
myself up and letting my third eye materialize
something on paper. This sustains me immeasurably!*

—MOTHER OF TWO CHILDREN,
age thirteen (twins)

*I take time for myself, exercise, play volleyball, or meet
friends for happy hour.*

—MOTHER OF A FOURTEEN-MONTH-OLD

*I actually LOVE football and have season tickets to the
Jets. My husband stays home (or my mom on days he*

can't) to watch the kids and I get to go to games and I
LOVE IT and that is all I need.

—*MOTHER OF THREE CHILDREN,*
ages six, four, and three

REPLACE PERFECTIONISM, WORRY AND SELF-CRITICISM WITH MINDFULNESS AND SELF-ACCEPTANCE

> *"Practice acceptance on yourself so you can be kinder*
> *with your child. Practice nonjudgmental awareness*
> *of your life so you can save your loved ones from*
> *the cruelty of your impossible standards and your*
> *hard-hearted disappointment. Practice greater faith*
> *and lesser blame."*
>
> —*Karen Maezen Miller, Momma Zen*

Another important aspect of taking care of yourself emotionally and mentally involves finding a level of acceptance within yourself and toward your children. Because, as hard as you might try, or whatever preconceived notions you might have about the kind of mother you will be and how respectful and well-behaved and well-adjusted your kids will be—*spoiler alert*—you will not be a perfect mother to your children, and your children will make their fair share of mistakes as well. Accepting that not everything will go according to plan, and that your journey as a mother will be just as much about letting go as about hanging on and trying to control, will better prepare you to ride the waves of motherhood with a smile on your face and in your heart. But from one who has seen some very dark, sad, anxious days as a mom struggling to stay afloat in the sea of perfectionism, I know my heart was most definitely not always smiling. I was, at times, one of the parents whom Wendy Mogel references in *Blessings of a Skinned Knee*: "I meet many parents who are trying so hard to be perfect parents, to make everything just right for their children, that they're draining away their pleasure in parenting.

They're too exhausted and too unconsciously resentful to enjoy the amazing show of childhood."

For moms to be able to find a deeper level of happiness in their lives, they need not only to be active fun-seekers but also to remember Richard Carlson's line, "don't sweat the small stuff." As a recovering perfectionist—"recovering" in the sense that my desire to be perfect (and my despair at not being perfect) never really goes away, but I continue to work on ways to constructively deal with it—I know how encumbered I have been over the past twenty years with "small stuff" regarding my children and myself as a mother. And boy, did I sweat! Just thinking of the countless hours and sleepless nights I spent worrying about the tiniest of blips that my children encountered, or "mistakes" that I made in parenting them, makes me wonder what I could have gotten done in that time—maybe I would be on my third book by now. But instead of being hard on myself for those "wasted" hours of worry, I would rather try to use my experience to encourage you to take a different path and to always keep your happiness in the forefront of your mind. (Note: there are situations where parents will most likely be very concerned about their children all of the time. If your child has a chronic illness, a disability, mental illness, or other issues that require extra time and thought to manage, your level of worry will naturally be higher than that of parents who are concerned with the more typical worries. Parents who shoulder life-and-death concerns about their children every day still need to work to care for themselves and to keep themselves emotionally strong and steady, although managing those types of worries is more about finding ways to live with the challenging situations, staying focused on the present, and managing the inevitable feelings of fear of what lies ahead.)

A guaranteed way to pull yourself out of the present moment and any possibility of feeling happy is to find something to worry about, or notice something "wrong" that you or your child are doing, and zero in on that. Just watch how quickly your smile turns to a frown and your brain begins to fill up with various forms of doom and gloom. In fact, according to a 2012 study published in the *Journal of Child and Family Studies*, more intensive forms of mothering correlate with worse maternal mental health.[23] The study examines what is known as the "parenting paradox," which refers to the fact that some mothers who describe their parenting role as being one of the most fulfilling roles of their lives *also* experience a great deal of stress and anxiety due to the intensity with which they parent, which in turn has a negative effect on their mental well-being. In an article on *Forbes.com* discussing the research, Alice Walton explains that "'intense parenting'—the belief that everything you do matters *sooo* much—might actually explain this 'parenting paradox' quite well. We all know an 'intense mother' when we see one (or perhaps we're intense parents ourselves), but the authors used five factors to encapsulate it well:

- *Essentialism* is the feeling that mothers, over fathers, are the more 'necessary and capable' parent.
- *Fulfillment* in parenting is defined by beliefs like 'a parent's happiness is derived primarily from their children.'
- *Stimulation* is the idea that you, the mother, should always provide the best, most intellectually stimulating activities to aid in your child's development.
- *Challenging* is, as you might guess, the idea that parenting is just about the most difficult job there is (participants ranked statements like, 'It is harder to be a good mother than to be a corporate executive').
- And *child-centered* refers to the idea that kids' needs and wants should always come before your own."

About 23 percent of the moms in this study were found to be depressed—which is much higher than the 6.7 percent of the general public who are depressed[24]—and this made the authors question why mothers are engaging in intensive parenting if it makes them unhappy. The study's authors conclude that women "may think that it makes them better mothers, so they are willing to sacrifice their own mental health to enhance their children's cognitive, social and emotional outcomes. In reality, intensive parenting may have the opposite effect on children from what parents intend."[25]

In other words, while mothers think they are doing something really good and important for their children by intensive parenting, they are actually stressed-out and unhappy—which in turn, as research has shown, can cause their children to become stressed-out as well (more on this in the boundaries chapter). My personal theory on why our society is in the throes of over-parenting has to do with the ways in which we were parented or not parented.

Many baby boomers and Gen X-ers who are raising kids today were themselves raised by parents who were far more detached and not nearly as hyper-focused on what we were doing as kids. Our parents did not know most of our teachers, were not involved in our homework or projects for school, and did not feel the need to make friends with all our friends' parents. They often did not know exactly where we were and could not easily get ahold of us (since there were no cell phones), and yet they did not seem overly bothered by this. We "kids", however, certainly remember what we were doing when our parents could not reach us—and this scares the hell out of us. So we hover and try to exert control to ensure that our kids will do things differently than we did. Well, lo and behold, in all of our helicoptering and controlling, we are unnecessarily stressing ourselves out and potentially not allowing our kids to be kids. And—another spoiler alert—despite our vigilante-type monitoring, our kids still sneak out and do some of the same stupid things that we did in high school, or so my twenty-year-old college sophomore recently informed me.

So, now that we may have the parenting paradox cleared up and understand that it is the *way* you parent, not the simple fact of being a parent, that can affect your level of happiness, it might be time to loosen up as you journey through motherhood.

Throughout all the challenges you will experience as a mother—whether you are managing a colicky baby, a highly sensitive toddler, a tween who has ADD, or a teenager who tells you for the first time that she hates you—remember that there is no "right" way to parent your children. You will find compelling books and articles about why you should medicate your child who has ADD, and just as many that will tell you that it is abhorrent to do so. You will find advice about how to tame your teenager, and articles about the importance of giving him space. So, you should absolutely do your research (knowing that you will often be even more confused), and then, ultimately, you should trust your instincts. Most importantly, do not be overly hard on your child or yourself. Know that you can always change the plan of action if Plan A doesn't work. As I tell my yoga students, "This is a yoga *practice*. There is no perfect. You just keep coming back to your mat again and again to work through things in your body and in your mind, and find new ways to move through challenging poses."

It is the same for parenting. We are not supposed to know how to do everything "right" with our kids. We try things. They try things. Sometimes things work and sometimes they don't. There is no perfect. We fail, they fail. They are learning how to function in the world, and are growing and changing every day. You will learn and grow along with your child, and do the best you can with the tools that you have. And if you feel that you are in way over your head, or truly do not know how to deal with some aspect of your child's behavior, make sure that you tap into your support system and get help. If you don't have a strong or reliable support system, consider finding some resources, like mothers' groups, to provide you with the support and feeling of connection that every mother needs. Most importantly, take care of yourself mentally and emotionally—every day. Walton reminds us, "It's so easy to feel that every little thing we do will have a make-or-break effect on our kids' development or success in life. But it's important to remember that this just isn't true. Putting our own mental health right up there with our kids'—

perhaps even first—is probably the best way to go. Since kids are so highly intuitive, working on [our] own happiness and mental health is the best thing we can do—though it's easier said than done, it's probably the best legacy we can leave."

COMPARE AND DESPAIR—
REPLACE JUDGMENT WITH COMPASSION

A friend of mine who moved here from another country when she was pregnant with her first child told me about the trouble she was having raising her "spirited" child. She says, "No one talks about how hard it is to be a mom. It seems like moms are always talking about how great their children are, but not about the struggles they have with them." She wonders whether this has been her individual experience because she is not from Minnesota and maybe just hasn't connected with enough moms at that deeper level, but she has a point. Many moms do feel alone in their "mom challenges" and are afraid to share the ugly truths about their children and themselves, especially when they look at Facebook and see how "happy" and "accomplished" every other kid on the planet is and how "easy" motherhood is for every other mother.

As many moms believe that they are expected to be able to "do it all" with a smile on their face, they can also easily feel as if they are falling short and sapping themselves of happiness, especially when they judge themselves by how their kids are faring or compare themselves or their children to others. When their kids struggle, some moms tend to get down on themselves for how they perceive themselves to be doing as mothers.

On the flip side, some moms are overly elated when their kids succeed, internalizing their children's accomplishments or good fortune as if they were their own. In other words, their happiness is based on the successes or failures of their children. Self-blame and self-aggrandizing are rampant among mothers. Does your daughter's perfect report card or your son's placement on the varsity soccer team make you feel happy? Of course. Are you sad that your daughter did not get placed in the advanced math class when most of her friends did? Sure. In both situations, do you look at yourself and ask yourself what you did right and what you did wrong? How much does this affect your overall level of happiness?

It is extremely important to understand early on that there will be many highs and lows with your children throughout their lifetimes, and that basing your level of happiness on these ups and downs is not recommended. I know this because there have been times in my parenting life—probably when I wasn't feeling so good about myself—when I have caught myself in that cycle, and it was not a healthy or happy place to reside. Of course you will be affected by your children's highs and lows (more on this in chapter 7), but your overall happiness needs to come from a deeper, more grounded, and secure place within you.

It is natural to assess how you are doing as a parent by how your child is doing, and when your child is not thriving or happy or well-adjusted, your heart will ache. Moms do have a hand in determining the kind of people their children become; however, in terms of judging yourself as a mother, it is important to examine the lens through which you are viewing yourself and to make sure that you are viewing both your child and yourself with compassion.

I accomplish this in part by noticing the simple moments, like when my thirteen-year-old son still lets me hug him in the hall at his school, even when his friends are around, or when my younger daughter walks in the door from school and gives me a sincere, ear-to-ear, *I love you and am so happy to see you* smile. We moms do feel proud of our kids for their tangible accomplishments, and we feel somewhat defeated when they have setbacks, but if you can look for the simple, heartwarming gifts that your children give you every day, it becomes much easier to find the happiness and joy in everyday mothering.

Another guaranteed happiness-zapper is the unfortunate underlying competition that exists between moms. Instead of supporting one another as they make their way through the murky waters of motherhood, there are some moms who secretly judge one another and compete against each other; they measure their own kids against their friends' kids or measure themselves against other moms. Here is a phrase I learned at the Emily Program: "compare and despair." Comparing yourself or your kids to others can bring you immediately to an unhappy place, or it can give you a false sense of happiness: "My kid is doing better than her kid." Yes, we all are guilty of passing judgment on other mothers and sometimes, as hard as we try not to, we look over our shoulders to see how we measure up to others.

But what every mother truly needs is the support and encouragement of other mothers. Most likely, you instinctively give this to your best friend, but remember that you should give it to other moms, even moms you don't know, as well. Like the mom whose three kids are being "*so* obnoxious" at the grocery store, throwing things out of the cart as quickly as Mom puts them in. You have a choice: you could walk right by this mom and think, *She must be a terrible mom to have such poorly behaved kids*, or you could take a more kind and compassionate approach by looking her in the eyes and saying with a smile, "Hey, it looks like the kids are winning—can I help you?"

She may decline your offer, with a hint of annoyance. Or she may burst into tears, thank you profusely and tell you how overwhelmed she is, that her husband has been out of town for two weeks, that she is at the very end of her rope, and that you just made her day—even her week. "And yes, please, I would *love* some help!" And each of you can walk out of the store feeling happy and good about yourself.

In the most simple terms, the best thing you can do for yourself and your fellow moms, in the common spirit and pursuit of happiness, is to do your best to find ways to lift each other up, instead of tearing each other down.

CHERISH THE MOMENT

For me, this is much easier said than done. I come from a long line of worriers. Worry must be etched deeply into my DNA. I distinctly remember the times when my grandfather would take all of us young grandchildren waterskiing in the summer, and my grandma would run into the cabin yelling, "I am going inside to have a heart attack!" We kids thought that was the funniest thing ever! We thought she was crazy and could not even fathom ever feeling like that. I didn't even really understand what she meant. I was way too busy laughing with my cousins, being a daredevil on water skis, having fun and enjoying life. Unfortunately, now I know exactly how my grandmother felt, and there are so many times when I want to run into the house (or just close my eyes) and scream the same thing as she did.

As I have mentioned before, I worry—not only when my kids do something risky, but also about how I am doing as a parent, about whether or not I am making the "right" choices for my kids when they are young, and making the right "suggestions" for them as they get older. The worry is almost like an old, worn-in, comfy sweatshirt that I cloak myself with, and which is covered in self-doubt and self-blame. But I continue to work on shedding that sweatshirt, or at least removing the "you are not good enough and therefore you are going to screw up your kids" mud stains. I really would like to ditch the worry sweatshirt altogether, but that may be almost impossible. I have yet to meet a mother who does not worry, at least a little bit, about her children.

What I have found, however, in my ongoing quest to lessen my levels of worry, is that focusing on the moment within yourself and with your children is a virtually fail-proof way to ward off perfectionistic and worrisome thoughts; it allows you to be more open to joy and happiness. That's because the moment is what is happening here and now. It is not about how things were, how they are "supposed" to be, how they will be, or how you or your kid screwed up or achieved some kind of greatness. Being present is simply being with what *is*, and finding acceptance of what is can lead to more happiness. It is not an easy place to allow yourself to be, given the hectic, frantically paced, worry-filled world we live in with our children, but the feeling of freedom and happiness that can be found in appreciating the beauty and wonder of the present moment can be almost magical. There is an ease and a levity that exists when you allow yourself to stay present and engaged in the moment. Being fully present in your life with your children is an immeasurable gift both for you and for your children, as it allows you to be better able to appreciate and embrace the time you have together—which, although it often does not feel this way when kids are young, truly is fleeting.

The most effective way to train yourself to be more in the moment is through breathing. By focusing on your breath for even one minute, you are immediately pulled into an awareness of your body and into the present moment. When you are in the car and stressed-out about traffic, all the bills you have to pay, or your kids screaming in the backseat, connect with your breath; this will slow down a racing heart or mind. There are CDs you can play in the car that guide you through breathing exercises (and would also be amazing for the kids) that can help you find your way from that just-about-to-lose-it feeling to a much calmer, more peaceful, happier place.

When you are at work, take a few moments during the day to place your hand on your belly and feel your breath to bring you into the present. Mediation is another great way to ground your mind and your body, release yourself from worry and anxiety, and allow yourself to be fully present. Even three minutes of quiet meditation before the kids get up in the morning can help you start your day in a more peaceful direction. There are times when I feel like all I do is race through my day, getting myself or the kids from one place to the next, checking off all the items on the to-do list. But breathing practices and regular meditation allow me to be better able to experience the joy around me and within. There is truly no time like the present.

◆ ◆ ◆

I don't know that any mother can fully grasp the "the days are long but the years are short" concept until she has experienced the exit of her eighteen-year-old child/adult, which, in my experience, feels like someone is ripping off one of your limbs. So, even on your most hellacious of days with your children, if you can remember that "this too shall pass" and that you truly have your children for only a blip of time—albeit a very, very important time of your life and theirs—it may allow you to find some brightness on a dark day. As I write this book, I am currently readying myself for the exit of child number two, and am in the midst of doing the "lasts" with him—his last birthday living in the house, watching him play his last high school basketball game, and soon his last high school baseball game . . . so I am knee-deep in nostalgia. I try to wrap my brain around the passage of time, and I try to grasp the reality of the idea that mothers pour every ounce of their hearts and minds into their children, only to have to let them go—whether or not they feel ready. And while many mothers are readily holding the door open for their child's exit, most moms—no matter how difficult their journey has been with their child—realize that this leg of the parenting expedition is over, which will cause them to wish they could go back and embrace the precious moments with their child a little longer. Anna Quindlen brilliantly shares her wisdom and feelings about wanting to hold on to time with her children in her essay "Good-bye Dr. Spock":

> *The biggest mistake I made is the one that most of us make while doing this. I did not live in the moment enough. This is particularly clear now that the moment is gone, captured only in photographs. I wish I had not been in such a hurry to get on to the next thing: dinner, bath, book, bed. I wish I had treasured the doing a little more and the getting it done a little less. Even today I'm not sure what worked and what didn't, what was me and what was simply life.*[26]

In truth, I have found that it is easier for me to discuss happiness, now that my children are pretty much self-sufficient. We all sleep through the night (unless I am waiting up for my teenager to come home); the diapers, potty-training devices, bottles, sippy cups, and car seats are gone, and my hip and shoulder are no longer numb from carrying the toddler that was basically an appendage of my body for a year. It's not that I was necessarily unhappy when I had young kids, but I did often feel suffocated by the demands of early motherhood. The other piece of feeling happier now is that I have the gift of experience. I now know that worrying about things, trying to control too many things with my children, and berating myself and/or my children if I do something *wrong* (perfectionism at its finest), destroys my ability to be happy. Now, I still have times when I do this to myself, and I can feel my happiness slip away. But I have learned that while no one is happy all of the time, I truly do deserve to be happy most of the time. I have learned that I am a better partner, friend, and mother when I put a stake in the ground for my own happiness, when I listen to the voice that says, "You are worth it," and ignore the one that says, "Hey you, who says *you* get to be happy? Remember, life sucks and then you die. Here, let me find something for you to worry about . . . "

So now, when I pull something out of my virtual happiness cup that I am excited to do, like meeting a friend for dinner, and my daughter cries and throws some guilt-inducing zingers my way because she wants me to help her with her homework, I give her a hug and a kiss and tell her I love her and that Daddy is the best homework helper in town, leave my guilt at the door, and make a mad, happy dash for my car. And other times, when my head is spinning because I have an article due or a presentation to prepare for or know I should really get to the grocery store, and I see that my son is looking at me and is definitely noticing the strained look on my face, I stop. I talk to him. I ask him how he is. I ask him if he wants to play a game or watch one of the funny videos he loves. Because in five years, this incredible son of mine, whom I love with everything I am, will be packing up his room and heading off to college. And in five years, I will still (I hope) be writing articles, planning events, and grocery shopping. But my son will not be sitting at the kitchen counter, staring at me with his gorgeous blue eyes and wondering if I am too busy or distracted to notice him.

The following veteran mothers share their advice and their hindsight about what they did or wished they had done to enhance their levels of happiness and joy while mothering their children:

What I would do differently is enjoy the little moments more. The quiet time snuggling, reading a book with them . . . I feel like I rushed through some of these moments because I was trying to be everything to everyone. Raising four kids it is hard to give them your undivided attention, but I would certainly, if given the chance, try harder to enjoy those special moments.

—MOTHER OF FOUR CHILDREN,
ages eighteen, sixteen, fourteen, and twelve

Definitely be more in the moment, worry less about all the things you need to get done. You get them done and then have to start over again. It's a never-ending cycle, so why not enjoy your moments more? Try to appreciate every stage along the way because you will not believe how fast time goes by. My advice for new moms would be to definitely not let yourself get consumed by your new mom role; it's okay to take time for yourself and in fact is very important for your sanity! Laugh a lot and know that each hard phase does pass by.

—MOTHER OF THREE KIDS,
nineteen, fifteen, and seven

The best advice I got was from a friend after a particularly awful morning with my three boys. I called her to tell her of how guilty I felt because I had spent the morning yelling and screaming at them to hurry up, pack up back packs, etc. I felt so badly that I sent them off to school with only screaming. She said to me, 'tomorrow is another day. You can do it better then.' That simple statement freed me from my guilt. Every day isn't perfect but kids get over it much quicker than we do and tomorrow is another day."

—MOTHER OF FOUR CHILDREN,
ages eighteen, sixteen, fourteen, and nine

Let your children see you having fun and enjoying life.

—MOTHER OF FIVE CHILDREN,
*ages twenty-six (twins), twenty-three,
twenty-one, and thirteen*

Kids don't need you to be perfect people. Kids need your love and your physical and emotional presence. They need your guidance and they need your respect. When you have a child, you are entrusted with the care of a fully formed soulful person. Souls are easily bruised and broken. Love, protect and nurture that soul to the very best of your ability. And open your own soul to the gifts that children bring.

—MOTHER OF TWO CHILDREN,
ages eleven and eight

Some other key components to combating perfectionism and increasing the joy in motherhood include the following:

◆ Take notice of your self-talk. Is it generally positive? Or is it more critical and negative? If it is negative, instead of trying to make the negativity go away, try to develop an oppositional voice that challenges the negativity. This is a voice that drowns out the negative voice of self-doubt and self-criticism and tells you that you can do it, that you are doing it, that you *are* doing the best you can, that you are the very best mother for your children.

◆ Shower not only your children, but yourself, with unconditional love. Always come back to the notion

that you are worthy of love and acceptance, even
when you make a mistake. This is an important
model for your kids to emulate.

◆ Seek levity (as in "lighten up") and work toward
releasing some of your emotional distress, which
is often caused by being unnecessarily critical of
yourself and your children. Do this by continually
looking for the "bright spot" within yourself and
them. Even when you are frustrated with their
behavior (or your own), try to think of Anne Frank,
who wrote, "Despite everything, I think people are
really good at heart."

◆ List the ways in which you express love, acceptance,
and compassion to your children and to yourself.

CHAPTER 6:

Self-Care Solution #4 — Find Gratitude and Connection

As mothers continually strive for a balance between taking care of their children, taking care of themselves, and finding happiness in all of it, one of the most proven and powerful methods of doing so is to connect with gratitude on a regular basis. As I discussed in the previous chapter, finding gratitude for the food you eat and for the ability to move your body every day can certainly provide you with regular doses of good feelings, but taking gratitude into as many aspects of your life as possible gives you a multitude of opportunities to stop, appreciate, and smile. Some moms are consistently able to feel gratitude for the special (and ordinary) moments they share with their children, and in their life in general. However, as Wendy Mogel explains in her book *Blessings of a Skinned Knee*, most moms are so bogged down with all of the responsibilities of motherhood, and their quest to do motherhood "right" or simply to get through the day, that they forget to look for or be open to seeing those moments. Many moms are somewhere in the middle, and will experience "time stands still" moments when their child first says "I love you," takes their first step, or reads their first word. Moms pause. Moms give thanks. Moms cry tears of joy and tears of gratitude and tears of "please, can we slow this whole thing down?"

But often those times of deep gratitude and pinch-yourself

moments are fleeting, because even before you wipe away your happy tears and realize that you've been smiling for a whole minute, real life kicks into high gear and there isn't time to stand around and emote because your to-do list is screaming at you, as is your other child, who desperately needs lunch and a nap. And furthermore, as if to balance out the joyous, pride-filled moments, moms often experience heart-stopping moments of a different breed—like those during which Mom is certain that she either is being *Punk'd* or is a participant on the show *Survivor*, due to the astonishing amounts of throw-up and diarrhea released from her child's body and deposited on her car, her bed, and a section of her brand-new living room couch.

But whatever type of moment, day, month, or year you are having with your children, it is important that you understand that connecting with gratitude in some way, every day, is an incredible way to smooth off the rough edges of motherhood and increase your level of happiness. Knowing that you won't feel grateful all the time as a mom, it is helpful to regularly make a concerted effort to step back and remind yourself of the gift of motherhood, as the following mothers do:

> *[Becoming a mother] changed me for the better in so many ways. The very best experience of my life— nothing will ever top being a parent. I am more patient, more caring, more spiritual, so many things I am grateful for in becoming a parent.*
>
> —MOTHER OF FOUR CHILDREN,
> *ages nineteen, sixteen, thirteen, and twelve*

> *Happiness is an emotion that comes and goes; no one is forever in a state of happy. Sometimes you are sad, afraid, worried, mad, and sometimes happy! I feel the key to happiness comes from being thankful, and I am very thankful for everything I have.*
>
> —MOTHER OF TWO CHILDREN,
> *ages eight and four*

From Oprah to *The Happiness Advantage* author Shawn Achor to Gretchen Rubin to Wendy Mogel to Robert A. Emmons, the world's leading scientific expert on gratitude, the power of gratitude and its relationship to happiness has been clearly identified. A November 2011 article on the Harvard Health Publications website states, "In positive psychology research, gratitude is strongly and consistently associated with greater happiness. Gratitude helps people feel more positive emotions, relish good experiences, improve their health, deal with adversity, and build strong relationships."[27]

Modeh ani are the first two Hebrew words of a prayer that observant Jews recite immediately upon waking, even before they get out of bed. The words are translated as "I give thanks." So the very first thing Jews are instructed to do when they open their eyes every morning is to say thank you—to thank G-d for being alive and for believing in him or her. There just has to be something to this—and there is, because I have tried it. I try to remember to say this prayer every day in my head when my alarm clock goes off and I so desperately want to close my eyes again and go back to sleep. But waking up every day and immediately connecting to gratitude for being alive is extremely powerful, and I would highly recommend it (and it does not have to be in the form of the Hebrew prayer; any acknowledgment of gratitude will do). I have found that gratitude can provide a sense of grounding, joy, and fulfillment, and that the more elements of gratitude I have incorporated in my life, the happier I've become. From finding gratitude on the yoga mat, to finding it through meditation, to exploring Judaism and all of its daily connections to gratitude through prayer and acts of kindness, I know for certain that I am happier when I am feeling and acting grateful.

There have been times during my motherhood journey, however, when I struggled to maintain any sort of meaningful connection to gratitude. In 2008, our family faced an extremely difficult financial blow coupled with the diagnosis of my father-in-law's pancreatic cancer; as I looked at our dwindling checking account and the bleak prognosis for pancreatic cancer patients, gratitude was certainly the furthest thing from my mind. In fact, looking back at how low I was during that time, I realize that it wasn't until I finally reconnected with hope and gratitude that, in spite of the pain I felt in dealing with the crises at hand, I started to pull myself out of my funk.

In an essay adapted from *Gratitude Works! A 21-Day Program for Creating Emotional Prosperity*, Robert Emmons speaks to the fact that gratitude is easy to find when life is just dandy, but when things feel like they are falling apart, it can feel almost impossible to wake up and say, "Wow, I am *so* thankful!" But Emmons says that we can and we must:

> *I have often been asked if people can—or even should—feel grateful under . . . dire circumstances. My response is that not only will a grateful attitude help—it is* essential. *In fact, it is precisely under crisis conditions when we have the most to gain by a grateful perspective on life. In the face of demoralization, gratitude has the power to energize. In the face of brokenness, gratitude has the power to heal. In the face of despair, gratitude has the power to bring hope. In other words, gratitude can help us cope with hard times.*[28]

Don't get me wrong. I am not suggesting that gratitude will come easily or naturally in a crisis. It's easy to feel grateful for the good things. No one feels grateful that he or she has lost a job or a home or good health, or has taken a devastating hit on his or her retirement portfolio.

But it is vital to make a distinction between *feeling* grateful and *being* grateful. We don't have total control over our emotions. We cannot easily will ourselves to feel grateful, less depressed, or happy. Feelings follow from the way we look at the world, the thoughts we have about the way things are and the way things should be, and the distance between these two points.

But being grateful is a choice, a prevailing attitude that endures and is relatively immune to the gains and losses that flow in and out of our lives. When disaster strikes, gratitude provides a perspective from which we can view life in its entirety and not be overwhelmed by temporary circumstances. Yes, this perspective is hard to achieve—but my research says it is worth the effort.

◆ ◆ ◆

In 2013, I had the incredible opportunity to travel to Peru on a Smile Network mission with three women friends to assist a team of doctors as they performed fifty-plus cleft lip and palate surgeries on children in need from all over the country. (Our assistance was non-medical, but sometimes we stood alongside them in the operating room.) During the five days we spent in the Lima hospital (which would not come close to passing code in the United States), there was hardly a moment when I was not completely filled with gratitude—gratitude that I could serve others, gratitude for my own health, for my family's health, for our access to health care, for living in America. And these mothers, oh my, they were some of the most incredibly grateful women I've ever met in my life. And their lives were hard—really, really hard—hard in a way that most of us will never know. But each one smiled—even when she had to wait nine hours with her child who was not allowed to eat or drink because of the *possibility* that she would be picked for surgery that day. And even when we told the mother that she would have to take her crying toddler home because the doctors were done operating for the day, she smiled—even though she knew that she would feed her child an evening meal and then start the fasting and the waiting all over again the next day. Was this her only hope for her child to have his lip or palate fixed? Probably. So of course all of the mothers would be grateful, right?

But I saw and felt something different in these mothers, something more than the fact that they were grateful because they had to be. I saw how gratitude kept their spirits alive. Because they had so little and expected so little, there was no taking anything for granted, and they could be truly and completely grateful for the smallest of things, like the "lucky" two-dollar bill that I gave to each one of them (which had actually been given to me by a generous friend to distribute). A few of the mothers, who had little or nothing material to give, and who had endured a great amount of heartache because many of their children suffered tremendously because of their cleft lips and palates— and, in some cases, other serious medical issues—brought me homemade gifts (a crocheted angel, a knitted scarf) because they wanted to express their gratitude by being able to give back.

I promised myself that in returning to the United States, I would do my very best to remember these women. And while I knew I would inevitably be caught back up in my day-to-day stresses, I have tried to keep this kind of broader perspective, and I truly have felt more grateful for the smallest of things—like air-conditioning (of which there was none in the children's hospital in Lima, when it was eighty degrees outside).

Gratitude is contagious. It spreads within you and fills you up with a sense meaning and groundedness. Gratitude makes you feel alive and connected to something much bigger than yourself. As author Melody Beattie writes her seminal self-help book *The Language of Letting Go*, "Gratitude unlocks the fullness of life. It turns what we have into enough, and more. It turns denial into acceptance, chaos to order, confusion to clarity. It can turn a meal into a feast, a house into a home, a stranger into a friend."[29]

I have also seen the effects of gratitude on my children. When my oldest son was going through a very difficult time in early teens, I was distraught. His grades were slipping, he was angry and belligerent at home, and I was extremely torn up inside with concern and worry—and of course I was asking myself, *What have I done wrong?* It was hard to reach him and hard to get him to be very agreeable about much of anything, but one thing that I insisted we do as a family on a regular basis was volunteer. Once every few months, I would gather everyone and we would head to a local food shelf and stock the shelves and pack bags for families in need, or, through the Minneapolis Jewish Family and Children's Service, we would deliver baskets and gifts to families in need on various holidays.

One night, on our way home from one of our volunteer shifts at the food shelf, he began to ask me questions like, "So, we didn't pack any fresh fruit or meat for the families, do they get any of that?" and "How long does that food we packed for them have to last them?" As I answered his questions honestly, I saw something in his eyes. Not only was it a deep compassion for the families in need that we served (who, he now understood, would eat most of their food out of cans and boxes), but it was also gratitude—gratitude for his life, for the fact that he would go home to a refrigerator full of fresh food, not having to ever worry about having enough to eat.

Another day, a cold day in December, I witnessed a bag of Hanukkah gifts transfer from my son's hands to those of an elderly Russian woman, who barely spoke a word of English but communicated through her eyes as they filled with tears of appreciation and joy. These experiences have been by far the best way to teach my children and myself the power of gratitude. And as my son matured and began to do more volunteer work through school—and ultimately began studying with an Orthodox rabbi who talked with him at length about the importance of gratitude—I saw a happy, self-assured, compassionate young man emerge. So I know firsthand that gratitude works.

GRATITUDE TIPS

- ◆ Count your blessings. Really. List them on paper. Revisit this list often and continue adding to it. A few ways to do this are:
  - *Keep a journal by your bed and when you wake up, write down three things you are grateful for.*
  - *Create a gratitude jar (Sean Achor's idea): every night or once a week, each member of your family writes down on a sheet of paper one thing they are grateful for and puts it in the jar. Periodically read the notes out loud to the whole family.*
- ◆ Tell people you care about that you are grateful for them. Tell your friends how much they mean to

you; tell your parents, kids, siblings, other family members and friends how much you appreciate them and why you do. You don't have to wait until someone's birthday or Father's Day or Mother's Day to express words of appreciation to someone. In other words, say thank you (and please), *a lot*. Find opportunities to thank your kids' teachers, bus drivers, and babysitters. When you thank the person who bags your groceries, your waiter at a restaurant, the checkout person at Target, look them in the eye and show them that you mean it. Not only will it make their day, but you will feel a more authentic, fulfilling connection to gratitude that makes you feel good as well.

◆ Take nothing for granted. Find gratitude in running water, electricity, air conditioning, heat, your car, your phone, education, health, and freedom. The more you can fill yourself up with gratitude, the more fulfilled and happier you feel.

◆ Give. One important way to feel and express gratitude is through giving. Giving feels good and helps you appreciate what you do have. Give of your time, your money, your energy to causes or people who need your help. Or even just giving a compliment, a smile, a nod, a hand to someone you know or to a stranger can be very powerful for both you and the other person.

◆ Try one of the gratitude websites or apps like Thankfulfor.com, Gratitude Journal for iPhone, or Gratitude Plus for iPad that help remind you to connect regularly with gratitude.

DIG DEEP—CONNECT WITH YOURSELF AND WITH OTHERS

Another critical component of self-care is the avoidance of avoidance. It is not running away from your troubles or secrets or shame. It is digging deep, through yoga, meditation, or the help of a trusted friend or counselor, to deal gently with your demons—emotional issues that hold you back from the freedom to be happy, freedom to care for yourself the way you know you want to. It is being sincerely and sometimes painfully honest with yourself, striving for self-awareness and authenticity, and dealing with your "stuff"—fear, anxiety, sadness, anger, shame—both the old repressed stuff and the new stuff. And instead of looking for the "great escape" in excessive food, exercise, shopping, a bottle of booze or pills, an extramarital affair, or anything that temporarily frees you from pain, worry, or stress, self-care means to strive continually to stay visible, aware, authentic, alive, and engaged within yourself and within the relationships in your life. Katie Arnold-Ratliff, articles editor of *O, the Oprah Magazine*, explains it like this:

> *Maybe you can experience levity enough to laugh, embarrassment enough to blush, irritation enough to bitch. But maybe the sadder, angrier, uglier stuff you drown out or deny. . . . But after a while you notice that you sure do watch a lot of TV, and change the subject all the time, and you're always ordering three whiskeys instead of one. You find that even your treasured relationships feel bloodless and rote . . . [and] you can't bear to be still because then you have to think.*
>
> *So, though it makes you sweaty with fear, you find yourself a shrewd therapist, and she cold-cocks you with this little number: 'Nobody gets to block out the bad stuff without losing the good.' You resolve to feel your feelings, starting with the big ones you've backlogged. . . . You see that you are strong enough to survive in the world and the hurt floating around in it. And you see that ditching an*

approach that . . . made you a stranger to yourself, left you only a partial person—feels really good.[30]

Having trusted friends and confidants with whom you can share your unfiltered feelings, your past and present hurts and joys, helps moms feel less alone in the often-confusing world of motherhood and womanhood. As is the case for many moms, I have found that, in raising my own children, some unresolved issues of my own childhood have resurfaced that I have needed to deal with. It is extremely common, when parenting teenagers, for memories of middle school and high school (the good, the bad, and the really ugly and embarrassing ones) that you had not thought of in decades to resurface. I am grateful that I have been able to turn to a few lifelong friends who "knew me when" to help walk me through some of these issues and offer their perspective to help me gain a better understanding of myself. These women (and sometimes men) can be honest mirrors in which you can check yourself. I have chosen my friends carefully. While I have many good friends and several different communities in which I am active (the Minneapolis Jewish community, my children's school community, the yoga community, the writing/blogging community), I have a handful of incredible people who truly know, understand, and respect the intricate workings of my heart and mind. I have trusted them with my deepest and darkest. And they have trusted me with theirs. They help me remix far too many old, destructive tapes that play in my head, and help me create new ones that are based on healthy belief systems based in compassion, acceptance, and self-love. They keep me grounded and real, and I try to offer them the same kind of love and acceptance that they offer me.

Developing and maintaining close friendships cannot be underrated. A huge component to practicing compassionate self-care is to connect thoughtfully with people who can be truly happy for your happiness, and concerned for your concerns. They will have an open shoulder for you to cry on and an open ear to listen to you, and they will know when to respond in an empathetic and loving way, when to offer constructive feedback, and when to just simply sit back and listen. And you will offer that to them as well. I have found that, as with many other aspects of self-care, nurturing friendships, old and new, will not just happen; it needs to be an intentional component of your self-care plan. According to Jessica Smock and Stephanie Sprenger, authors of *The HerStories Project: Women Explore the Joy, Pain, and Power of Female Friendship*, the bonds of "women's friendship can be just as intimate as marriage and essential to emotional health."[31]

STRATEGIES FOR CONNECTING WITH OTHERS

- ◆ Join a neighborhood or community playgroup to connect with other moms.
- ◆ Join a local gym or a running, biking, or walking club where you can have regular contact with other women.
- ◆ Rekindle some relationships with old friends. Reach out to your old high school bestie, even if has been ten years since you last connected.
- ◆ Get to know the parents of your kids' friends. Invite them over for a cup of coffee while the kids run around outside, or invite their whole family for a meal.
- ◆ Volunteer. There are so many ways to volunteer in the community, at your church or synagogue, or at your children's school—and what a great way to meet good-hearted people.
- ◆ If you work, reach out to other mothers in your place of employment so that you have trusted people to talk to at work.
- ◆ If you really feel that you have "no time" to devote to friends, reach out to moms online. With the Internet and social media at our fingertips, we could not be in a better position to find the support, understanding, and morale boosters we need as mothers. Find blogs that you like and join online moms' groups.

WHAT IF YOU ARE NOT HAPPY?

Even when you are intentional about trying to practice self-care, sometimes life as a mother can still feel extremely overwhelming. As you experience the ups and downs that are consistent with motherhood and with life in general, it is important to be keenly aware when negative, depressed, or anxious feelings are taking over your psyche and you just can't shake them. Some women are blasted with this right out of the motherhood gates, when postpartum depression throws a wrench into everything they thought new motherhood would be like. Some moms experience some type of depression a little later as sleep deprivation and the incredible demands of new motherhood leave them feeling like a dark cloud has landed on them and they don't know how, when, or if they will feel like themselves again. And other mothers feel the weight of depression when their children are older and they experience the hormonal changes of perimenopause and menopause. Nonetheless, all mothers nod in unison when reading this statement from Alice Walton on *Forbes.com*:

> *Parenthood might just be one of the most psychologically challenging enterprises there is. Almost any parent will agree that the indescribable joys can be matched by equally intense feelings of worry, doubt, helplessness, anxiety, and, of course, depression. This is the great 'parenting paradox' that psychologists (not to mention parents) have pulled their hair out over.*

Sometimes it is hard to know when unhappiness is situational (or "just a stage") and when it is a more longstanding, serious mental health issue that needs professional attention. You undoubtedly will be exhausted as a new mother, you will most certainly feel down when and if your child is going through a tough time, and your kids are almost guaranteed to throw you regular curveballs as you attempt to create happiness in your home and within yourself. A wonderful dinner that you spent all day preparing could end up being the impetus for a full-blown power struggle between you and your strong-headed toddler who refuses to even take one bite, leaving you both in tears. A much-anticipated family outing at the zoo (which is an hour away from home) could turn sour when your "potty trained" three-year-old has an unexpected accident and you had decided not to pack extra clothes because he hasn't had an accident in three months. Teenagers are infamous for throwing a wrench into many best-laid plans, with their sometimes (or often) resistant and rebellious attitudes and behavior, and they can deplete you of every ounce of your parenting reserve tank, leaving you feeling totally spent, frustrated, and sometimes unhappy.

When you find yourself experiencing what seems to be situational depression or a circumstantial funk, it is important that you go back to the happiness check-in questions and also pull up your list of happiness boosters. I needed to be very diligent about practicing yoga and spending time with women friends (and if not in person, then by phone) when my two older kids went through some of their most hellacious times during middle school. I was sad, scared, anxious, and just plain down when dealing with the pain and frustration that each of them felt when they were bullied or excluded, or when they acted in ways that made me wonder if I had done something terribly wrong in raising them. When I did not do the things that grounded me during these stressful times, I became emotionally overwhelmed, which felt awful and certainly was of no help to my children. And there have been other times over the past twenty years when my kids were doing great, but I was down because my husband and I were completely off balance, or because I simply could not find the happy place within myself. These are the times when you truly need to be proactive about your mental and emotional well-being, and to be very honest with yourself about what you need to "lighten your load" and infuse yourself with more joy.

During times when you do feel "off," it is essential for you to give yourself little lifts to shake things up in a good way. As a mother of three I interviewed advises, "Find something you love to do and do it as often as possible." Whether it is a small, relatively easy thing you can incorporate into your life—like getting silly with your children, reconnecting with your best friend from grade school, making new friends, attending church or synagogue, joining a book club, starting guitar lessons, taking a cooking class, writing in a journal, mindfully focusing on the positives in your life instead of the negatives, and/or borrowing some of the happiness boosters from the mothers earlier in this chapter—or more complicated moves, like changing jobs or exiting an unhealthy relationship, make sure that you are continually, mindfully and compassionately doing what you need to do for yourself to keep joy alive within you.

If you are at a place, however, where the things that used to provide you with a strong shot of happiness to carry you through the day, week, or month are no longer working, and you find yourself irritable, moody, withdrawn, sad, and lethargic, then it is important that you be honest with yourself and consider seeking help. Many mothers, during various stages of their motherhood journey, become depressed or anxious and need some type of therapy and/or medication. For me, even before I ended up at my sister's doorstep, I knew something was really wrong as I often found myself at the end of a yoga class, lying in *savasana* (corpse pose) with tears rolling down my face—and then leaving the class, which had always provided me with just the right ratio of grounding to uplifting, feeling down in the dumps.

I had been relatively diligent about checking in with a therapist when I felt I needed a "tune-up," and I would usually leave those sessions feeling lighter. However, I noticed that for close to a year, there was little that could ease the heaviness I felt inside. I noticed my son asking me why I was sad all the time. I felt guilty for flying off the handle with my teenage daughter more often than necessary. I was snappy with my husband and somewhat withdrawn socially. I developed an almost debilitating fear of speaking in public, even in simple, non-threatening situations like introducing myself at a meeting, and had several panic attacks on airplanes. As a yogi and a very health-conscious person, I had been opposed to taking mood-altering medication;

I did not want to become dependent on a pill for my happiness or ease. However, after much research and many hours of discussion with my therapist, close friends, family members, and my husband, I decided that I did indeed deserve to be happy and that I had tried everything and anything that I thought could help free me from the anxious and depressive state that I was stuck in.

In using the motto that I developed during my recovery from the eating disorder, and understanding that the anxiety and depression was a chemical issue rather than something I could control, I made the decision about the medication: I chose life. Which, for me, meant giving an antidepressant a try. And thankfully, after a month of feeling like I was literally crawling out of my skin, it worked. I remember the moment: I was driving in my car with my daughter in the backseat, and just daydreaming, thinking about nothing in particular. My daughter said something silly and she laughed. And then I laughed—*really* laughed. And I realized that this subtle yet powerful feeling that was filling up my entire being—a feeling that, until that simple moment of laughing with my daughter, I had not realized how much I had missed—was happiness.

From that moment on, I have not taken happiness for granted. I try my best to treasure and honor it and actively seek out ways to create it, feel it, and give it to others. And even though I was able to wean myself off of the medication after about eighteen months, I have developed a great appreciation for the fact that these types of medications exist, and can truly help people with situational or ongoing depression or anxiety. I would not hesitate to use this medication again if I felt that my grip on happiness was slipping out of my hands, nor would I judge anyone else for using medications like this one. I love the honest self-assessment by Kim Brooks, in her article for *Salon* entitled, "Is Motherhood Causing My Depression?" in which she talks her about her ongoing battle with depression, her unsettled feelings about being a SAHM (or stay-at-home mom—more on this in chapter 9), and her questions about her use of medication: "I think the issue is more that for some women, women like me—with a history of depression and a hereditary predisposition toward emotional instability—motherhood and sanity just aren't 100 percent compatible."

BE MINDFUL OF HOW YOU
FILL UP YOUR HAPPINESS CUP

Speaking of sanity, another important factor to be aware of as you seek happiness in your life is the coping and self-soothing mechanisms you employ to deal with the stresses of motherhood. Whether it is shopping, smoking, exercising, eating, or drinking, any vice that is used to numb yourself from the strain (or in some cases, boredom or monotony) of motherhood can end up being destructive if not kept in check. A May 2013 *Psychology Today* blog post discusses a study by Caron Treatment Centers, conducted that same year,[32] which outlines the top five reasons moms turn to alcohol and drugs: "stress or anxiety, romantic relationships, pressure from family or friends, traumatic experience and a general feeling of boredom."[33] It is essential for moms to acknowledge if and when they cross over from drinking socially to needing a drink (or five) to get through the day.

According to an April 2014 *TODAY Parents* article entitled "Hitting the Mommy Juice Too Hard? Experts Warn of Alcohol Abuse by Moms," almost 40 percent of respondents to a TODAY. com survey "said drinking helps them cope with the stress of being a parent and more than one-third said they have mom friends who they think have a problem with alcohol." The article reports that wine is the preferred beverage and that "companies have noticed, creating wine brands targeting stressed-out moms, with names like Mad Housewife, Mommy's Time Out and Mommy Juice. Sales are up 25 percent."[34]

Now, don't get me wrong, I love going out with girlfriends and losing myself in conversation, laughter, and hearty helpings of pinot noir; however, because of my addictive personality, there have been times when I have needed to ask myself whether pouring myself a glass of wine as I am making dinner is the best idea. Sometimes my answer is yes, and sometimes I opt to call a friend instead (and occasionally we have glass of wine together over the phone). But whatever I decide, I try to be honest with myself about how I am feeling and what I need to do to take care of these feelings and my whole self in a healthy and constructive manner. Whatever tactics you enlist to create happiness in your life and manage the stress of motherhood, make sure that you are aware that, just as the media and marketers prey on women with their sometimes-unhealthy messages about body image, diet, and exercise, they also do this with the allure of alcohol. It may serve moms better to think of the 1970s slogan "Calgon, take me away" (as in taking a bath with Calgon bubbles to relieve stress) rather than thinking that mommy needs to escape by drinking her "Mommy Juice."

It is critical to remember that your level of happiness comes from the inside, in allowing yourself to connect with others in a meaningful way. Relying on sources like alcohol, food, or clothing or money to *make* you happy will keep you in an ongoing spiral of dependency, and ultimately will stand in your way of being truly peaceful and contented.

As Helen Keller reminds us, "Happiness cannot come from without. It must come from within. It is not what we see and touch or that which others do for us which makes us happy; it is that which we think and feel and do, first for the other fellow and then for ourselves."

CHAPTER 7:

Self-Care Solution #5 — Set Boundaries

When they were very small, I suppose I thought
someday they would become who they were because of
what I'd done. Now I suspect they simply grew into
their true selves because they demanded in a thousand
ways that I back off and let them be.

—*Anna Quindlen*, Loud and Clear

It was my three-year-old son's first day of preschool. I confidently walked him into the synagogue and down the hall to his classroom, feeling his small hand gripping mine tightly. As we approached the door, I glanced down at his face and saw his eyes fill with that familiar look that said, "You are not really going to leave me in this joint, are you?" My heart filled with a bit of dread but I held his hand tighter and opened the door.

Upon entering the already noisy room that bustled with moms and their toddlers, and which smelled of animal crackers and apple juice, I gathered up some toys and sat down with him, hoping to engage him in an all-consuming activity that would distract him from my impending departure. He was completely taken in by the rumbling sound the toy truck made as he intently pushed it back and forth on the blue carpet. I seized my opportunity and gingerly stood up and headed for the door. One step away from the door, I heard him start to whimper. I turned to look at him (BIG, HUGE no-no!), and I saw the tears pooling in his eyes and his lower lip quivering. Willing myself to go numb, I opened the door ever so slightly and shimmied out of the room, quickly closing the door behind me. As the door clicked, the volume and intensity of his cries increased dramatically and I could hear his shrieks and gasps for breath as I walked down the hall toward the synagogue exit. I stopped dead in my tracks and as if on cue, one of the teachers poked her head out of the room and said, "He will be fine. Really, he will be."

Avoiding the gaze of other moms coming in and out, I shuffled out of the building, got into my car, and dropped my head onto the steering wheel. My whole body shook as I felt his sadness and fear permeate my body and mind, his tears blending into mine. This was my baby boy, and I had been looking forward to having a little time to catch my breath: a few hours a week to write, to sleep, to walk, to go to Target by myself, or just to think.

My head felt like a dead weight against the steering wheel.

I didn't want to move. I told myself that I would wait ten minutes, and then go back in to make sure he was okay. My heart raced, my mind spun. I questioned myself. "What am I doing? I don't really need to be doing this. I have committed to being a stay-at-home mom for now. Maybe I am being selfish wanting this time for me. But I know that this will be good for him. He needs to socialize with other kids, to be away from me for a little while. I hope he is okay. I hope he stopped crying, I hope he is sitting by one of his buddies, eating animal crackers, and that his teacher will give him a ball (did I tell the teacher that he is obsessed with balls?), and that he is fine. He will be fine, right? I will be fine. I should just leave. But what if he is not fine? I don't think I am fine."

This conversation continued inside my head for a few more minutes until I opened my car door and walked slowly back into the building and down the hall to his classroom. My ears soon filled with the sound of his wails. I approached the door, peeked into the one-way glass cutout above it, and saw him literally plastered against the door, pulling away from the teacher who was gently trying to peel him away from his escape route. His screams,

"MAAAMMMAAA, MAAAMMMMAAAAA!" pierced my ears and my heart. Ignoring the voice of reason in my head saying, "He will be okay . . . it just takes time to adjust . . . go back to your car and drive away," I opened the door, picked up my tear- and snot-drenched son, turned to the teacher and said, "I don't think this is going to work for us." I closed the door and walked out of the building, wrapping my unglued son in my embrace, hoping that my arms would help to glue him back together.

To this day, I don't know if I made the right decision to wait another year to send my son to preschool, and I would deal with an even more agonizing decision years later when I decided to give my youngest daughter, a preemie and a late-spring birthday, an extra year in school. But this pattern of putting my children before myself would continue, and there were times when I felt that I could never, ever do enough to protect them from the inevitable pain of life. As almost every mother will attest in regards to her own life, in attempting to appease my children I often did not choose what was best for me. Setting clear boundaries is by far my weakest area as a mother, as separating myself from my children mentally, emotionally, and sometimes physically has been a battle within myself that I feel I often lose. I feel my children's feelings, and I take on their issues as if they are my own. I struggle—I mean I *really* struggle, at a cellular level—to understand where I stop and they start, or where they stop and I start. I continually battle my feelings: *Did the decision I made for them mess them up forever? What if I make a mistake? What if that popular piece of advice, "trust your instincts," sometimes leads me into a spinning frenzy in which I want to yell, "What if I just don't know?" What if my instincts change and what I thought was 'right' at one time, I now think may have been 'wrong'?*

Many moms I interviewed also admitted to taking on way too many of their children's emotions in an effort to try to save them from having to feel sad, disappointed, defeated, or rejected—emotions that all human beings will encounter at some point in their lives and will need to know how to process. Not only is this unhealthy for the mother, but if moms continue to try to "make it all better" for their children, how will children learn to self-soothe and deal with negative emotions? They most likely will not develop these necessary coping skills, and it will become even harder to develop them as they get older.

It is impossible to know how and when obstacles will come up for your children, and you certainly can't predict when they will stumble, how they will recover, what will throw them off track, and what will make them stronger. Still, knowing where to draw the line between your children's emotions and your own is essential for both your well-being and that of your children. It takes insight and a keen awareness of boundaries to determine how much to get involved your children's lives, when to back off, and when to push them.

When I once asked my dad for advice about a problem one of my kids was having, he replied with one of his favorite lines: "Just let him be—he'll figure it out." I agree with this message to a certain point. But there were times as a kid when I longed for more guidance and emotional support, even when I acted like I didn't need it. So, as a parent, I have done quite a bit of overcompensating, as many of us Gen Xers have, and tend to err on the side of over-involvement. Sometimes this has worked and sometimes it has backfired, and I am still working every day within myself and with each one of my kids to figure out where those boundaries are. I have found that it is rarely crystal clear and it is certainly not easy.

The helicopter generation makes self-care in terms of setting healthy boundaries extremely challenging. Having 24/7 access to children with cell phones and apps that allow moms to find out where their kids are and what they are doing at almost all times lures mothers to hover in their children's business. And even if you are not doing so, it sometimes can feel like you are doing something wrong because of these types of scenarios:

> **Charlie to his mom:** "Joey's mom texted him four times during the sleepover at Jimmy's. You didn't text me at all. You don't care about me!"

Joey to his mom: "Mom! You are so overprotective! Charlie's mom didn't text him at all when we were at Joey's! Why can't you back off and let me be?"

It sometimes feels like you can't win. The most important thing is to talk about expectations with your children, and to remember that even though "all the other moms" are doing it a certain way, you need to take care of yourself. If you are texting your child during his sleepover while you are having a date night with your partner, you are not allowing yourself to fully let go and be in the moment.

◆ ◆ ◆

I had the privilege of hearing Wendy Mogel speak at an event, and when she signed my copy of her book *Blessings of a B-*, which had become a source of guidance and inspiration to me, I was able to pose one quick question to her. It was in regard to a statement made by a mother I had surveyed, and repeated to me by my mother-in-law on several occasions: "Do you believe the saying that you are only as happy as your saddest child?"

Her reply was simple, straightforward, and instantaneous. "Absolutely."

I didn't know if I should feel validated or deflated. There is no question that mothers feel their children's pain at their core. However, if Wendy and I had had more time to chat, I have a feeling that she would have gone on to remind me—as she discusses in her book—that it is important for moms to make healthy, real attempts to detach from the roller coaster of emotions that our children will go through during their years with us (and after), so that we are able to properly care for ourselves and those we love.

Trying to shield your children from life's inevitable pains is exhausting work, and I have spent an inordinate amount of time and energy trying to do so. What I often lost sight of, in my attempts to shield them from pain, was the pain that I endured in trying to make everything okay for them (and "making everything okay" is, of course, impossible). Through many years of trial and error, I have realized that trying to absorb the uncomfortable stuff in their lives so they don't have to has been unhealthy for both them and me. I realized that an underlying reason for my struggle to separate and detach a bit (or *a lot*) from my children was because I was unable to draw protective boundaries around myself to allow me to be me, to take care of my own needs while also catering to the needs of my family. In order to become better at doing so, I needed to practice all the self-care tactics mentioned in this book, and to continue to connect on a daily basis to this quote from the Talmud (the body of Jewish civil and ceremonial law and legend): "If I am not for myself, then who will be for me? And when I am for myself, then what am 'I'? And if not now, when?"[35]

The clinical term for having difficulty separating one's self from another is *enmeshment*, and it can easily happen in parenting. According to *Dr. Margaret Paul, coauthor of Do I Have to Give Up Me to Be Loved by You?*, "Enmeshed parenting describes a style of parenting that can cause problems in your child's successful development of their own personality, ethics, and values. There are a number of signs and symptoms to look out for to determine if you may be an enmeshed parent:

- ◆ Your children's good or difficult behavior, and successful or unsuccessful achievements, define your worth.
- ◆ Your children are the center of your life—your sole purpose in life.
- ◆ Your entire focus is on taking care of your children, rather than also taking care of yourself.
- ◆ Your happiness or pain is determined solely by your children.
- ◆ You are invasive—you need to know everything about what your children think and do."[36]

As you can probably tell by now, I can identify with every single one of those points. I do believe that most mothers can relate to at least of few of these to a certain extent, but the key to maintaining healthy boundaries is to stay connected with who *you* are, separate from your children. In an effort to take an honest look at your level of enmeshment with your children, and to remind yourself about the importance of boundaries, consider the following questions:

- On a given day, tally up the number of minutes or hours in a day you worry about your children.
- Does worry about your children keep you up at night?
- Is the worry propelling you to act, or are you simply spinning in the worry?
- On a scale of one to ten, how much does your child's mood affect you?
- When your child experiences disappointment or failure, how does that feel to you and how do you handle these feelings?
- When your child comes to you with a problem, what is your first inclination?
- On a scale of one to ten, how strong is the urge for to you want to fix your child's mistakes or problems?
- What does it feel like if you try to NOT fix them?
- How often do you experience guilt in relation to your children (i.e. when you miss a soccer game or choir concert, or if they cry when you leave them alone)?
- How often does this guilt prevent you from doing things away from your children?

Once you have answered these questions, you will probably have a good sense of how you are doing in the boundary department. In the following sections, we'll talk about how to define the concrete physical and emotional boundaries that are an essential aspect of your self-care prescription. Every mom has to determine for herself what her specific need for physical and emotional space looks like, but whatever your criteria are, it is crucial that you are continually aware of drawing healthy lines between yourself and your children in an effort to steer yourself clear of enmeshment parenting.

PHYSICAL BOUNDARIES

The moment you became a mother, your sense of self and your idea of personal space were forever changed. An embryo starts out by occupying a tiny space in your uterus, and you pray that these cells will grow and develop into the baby you've been dreaming of. Then she is eight pounds and you feel like you are suffocating and there is NO more room in your belly and you need to get her out—and disconnect her from your body—*now!* And then she is attached to your breast (if you're nursing) and to your body as you carry her around, and you dream about times when you can just put her down and walk out of the room for a moment without her crying. Your bedroom is no longer the private and sacred space that you and your partner once shared. It is a place where the baby often resides, whether in your bed or close by in a bassinet—or maybe she is down the hall, but the baby monitor (which projects her every breath and every cry) is set in front of (and blocking) the candles and massage cream on your nightstand.

Babies, toddlers, and children take up physical space as well—a lot of it. Their stuff takes up square footage in your home. And just when you have gotten over tripping over their toy cars in the living room, they are begging to use your parking space in the garage ("Please, just for tonight because it's going to be *freezing* in the morning when I leave for school!") They take up a space in your bank account (but that is a chapter unto itself), and they take up space in your heart and in your mind. Looking back at your tear-stricken, pleading five-year-old one more time (even though you promised yourself you were just going to keep looking straight ahead as you left his kindergarten classroom on the first day of school) is enough to make you feel as though you have been stabbed twenty times in the heart, and you vow to quit your job and homeschool your children until they graduate high school.

Fast-forward thirteen years: as you are packing up your daughter for college, you feel the sudden urge to plead with her to stay with you for just a little longer (or maybe you can't get her out the door fast enough!). This push-pull is constant; you want to keep them close, and you also want—and need—to push them out of the nest so they can fly on their own. And while you are going through these push-pull cycles, they are individuating and feeling their own urges to keep you close and also push you away. Throughout it all, your need for your own space will be challenged. But you must find a way to create and preserve it.

Your space can be anywhere. If you work outside your home, it can be your office or cubicle. If you work at home (whether as a stay-at-home-mom or at a paying job), could you create some space of your own in your house or apartment? It does not need to be a fancy, high-tech, spacious office, just a place in your house that you can call your own. It can be a tiny little corner in any room where you can put a small desk or a round table and a chair. But it is a space that requires clear boundaries, an invisible (or visible) sign that says "mom's space."

As a writer, I have always craved a dedicated writing space. When I worked for *Momtalk* magazine, I would go to the company's corporate offices so I could focus on completing articles or editing the magazine. I found that when I tried to work from home, without a defined workspace, it was too easy to get distracted with laundry, dishes, cleaning, the phone, etc. We had a small, well-lit, unused area in my home that I dreamed of making into an office for years. And now here I sit, in my writing haven that is filled with natural sunlight and *my stuff*—my favorite books, photo albums, keepsakes and, most importantly, my writing desk. When I am in this space, I feel peaceful and connected to myself in a way that I don't feel anywhere else. I feel inspired to write, to think, to create, and to breathe freely. When I leave this physical space, I try to keep the idea of this space with me as my thoughts become cluttered with everyone else's stuff—whether it's my kids', husband's, friends', or family's.

As Kate Hopper, author of *Ready for Air* and *Use Your Words:*

A Writing Guide for Mothers, told me: "After a couple of years of me spreading my stuff out on the dining room table, my husband had had it, and he turned the tiny pantry off our kitchen into an office for me. It's small and cluttered, but it's mine. Another writer friend turned an even smaller closet into an office and she loves it in that tiny space."

Creating a physical space of your own can be symbolic of creating and protecting a space within yourself. There have been times when something upsetting has happened to one of my kids, and I have become so overcome with worry or frustration that I felt like I "lost myself." When that happens, I try to center and ground myself through meditation and yoga, in an effort to create the healthy space I need to be able to tap into my own spirit and my own sense of self that is separate from my children.

As you work to define physical and emotional boundaries with your children, know that this is an ongoing process and one that will involve a continual feeling of push/pull. Sometimes your children will want to pull you close in, and other times, they will try to kick you to the curb. Sometimes you cannot help yourself from getting pulled into their emotional lives, wanting to protect them from harm. The following questions will help you explore the difficult and ongoing question that all mothers ask when attempting to foster a healthy relationship with their children: "For my own self-preservation, where do I draw the line?"

- ◆ Do you have a space in your home that is your own?
- ◆ Where do you go when you need a mental or physical break from your children? If a room or part of a room in your house isn't possible, how about a park or a coffee shop?
- ◆ How do you feel when you don't get enough space for yourself?
- ◆ How do you feel when you do?
- ◆ How much alone time do you need?
- ◆ How much do you get?

♦ Are you able to ask for help from others to get some time alone?

TIPS FOR DEFINING PHYSICAL BOUNDARIES
♦ If at all possible (even if it is a corner of a closet), create a "room of one's own" in your home that represents:
  • *A place that you can retreat to when you need a break*
  • *A place where only your stuff belongs*
  • *A place where the kids' stuff does not pile up*
  • *A place where you can leave a piece of paper and know that it will be there when you return*
  • *A place where you can gather your thoughts and connect with yourself*
  • *A space that is clearly defined to yourself, your partner, and your children*
♦ Be aware of when you need to separate yourself physically from your children. Notice when you feel your emotions escalating to very high levels, when you feel that you may do or say something to your child that you know you will regret. In that event:
  • *Leave the room.*
  • *Walk away.*

Find a space that is separate from your children where you can take a deep breath and settle yourself down (maybe it is just the next room over, or maybe it is "your space" that you have created). Nothing constructive happens when you are dealing with your child from a heightened, emotionally charged place. This is also a time when I look at myself closely and ask: How much sleep have I gotten in the last twenty-four hours? Is something else upsetting me that is contributing to my short fuse?

EMOTIONAL BOUNDARIES
I remember the feeling vividly. It started as a physical sensation; oftentimes it happened when I was nursing one of my babies, or

when one of them had fallen asleep on my belly and I could not feel where my body stopped and hers started. Each one of her breaths and beats of her heart morphed into mine—I was her and she was me. And in the beginning, this felt good. The physical and emotional connection to my child, my flesh and blood, made me feel like I was a more complete version of myself. It also gave me a sense of power—I knew her just as well as she knew herself and I could protect her from any and all pain. But inevitably, over time, it became clear that this power was not real, and this sense of "oneness" that I felt became problematic and unhealthy, as the lack of emotional boundaries between my children and me made it confusing for me to sort out what was my "stuff" and what was theirs. I found myself feeling so terrified that they would experience pain and confusion, to the extreme level that I did as a child and an adolescent, that the generalized worry I carried around felt like a thousand-pound weight attached to my heart. Often I would also throw in a paralyzing fear that doing something "wrong" in parenting my kids would result in catastrophic consequences for them. These kinds of thoughts and fears have often created so much internal pressure that my levels of anxiety have skyrocketed, as in the case that I outlined in the introductory chapter. And even though I continue to slip and fall in this area of self-care, I have realized (again, with the help of therapy, yoga, and meditation) that for moms to practice self-care at a deep emotional level, they need to be continually aware of and compassionate toward the flurry of the emotions that arise when they are parenting their children. Allowing yourself to feel and grapple with your own emotions (many of which will appear out of nowhere and arise when you least expect them), as well as allowing your child to feel and grapple with his or her own emotions (which is sometimes brutally painful), are the most critical components to defining your emotional boundaries with your children.

As I parent my own children, I have made a strong effort to help them develop their emotional intelligence, and to establish their emotional boundaries, by encouraging them to be aware of their feelings and the feelings of others, and to trust themselves to use their voice to express their feelings. I try to ask them how they feel about certain situations before sharing my feelings or opinions with them. One night, after a dinner out with our extended family, my nine-year-old received an impromptu invitation to sleep over at her grandparents', which she often does like to do. Our whole family was looking at her to see how she would respond. I saw her chin drop to her chest and her eyes lower. Instead of jumping in to "rescue" her, I let her connect with her feelings so she could be the one to make and voice her decision. She lifted her head back up and looked at me and whispered in my ear, "I don't really want to go tonight but I feel like people are going to be mad at me if I don't." I told her that it was perfectly fine to thank her grandparents for the invitation and say that she would like to sleep over another night, but not tonight. So that is what she did.

And there it was—her inner voice, her truth, her voice of self-care and self-advocacy—and I was thrilled that my daughter had enough self-awareness and confidence to assert her feelings as well as her fears of letting people down. This is the exact voice that I am still working to cultivate for myself, and the voice that all mothers continually need to listen to and respect as we pour our hearts and souls into raising our children and caring for our families. This is the voice that tells us that if we are truly going to be able to care for those we love, we need to start by caring for ourselves.

TIPS FOR DEFINING EMOTIONAL BOUNDARIES

- ◆ Be compassionate and empathetic toward your children, but remember that you need not be the built-in shock absorber for their joy, pain, or discomfort.
- ◆ Take note of how you feel when your child is in pain, anxious, sad, afraid, or mad. Try to separate out what is actually yours and what is theirs. Remind yourself that it is not only okay for your child to feel these

feelings, but necessary so she can develop the tools to deal with them. Resist the urge to try to take on these feelings "for" your child; instead, encourage her to talk about *her* feelings and help her deal with them in a constructive manner.

◆ Address your level of worry. When you find yourself worrying about your child, ask yourself these important questions:
  - *Is the worry producing any positive changes for your child, or for you?*
  - *Are you truly concerned about your child's well-being, or are you concerned about yourself and how your child's actions or inactions are affecting you or will reflect upon you?*
  - *Can you turn your worry into action?*
  - *Can you find a way to let it go by talking through it with a friend, therapist, or spiritual advisor?*
  - *Do you think you would describe worrying about your children as a habit?*
  - *If so, what tactics can you use to break or at least reduce the habit? (Try meditation, yoga, or breath work.)*

◆ Deal with guilt.
  - *When you find yourself spinning in a guilt storm relating to something you did or didn't do for your children, develop new thought patterns that start with the following statements: "I am a loving and caring mother and I am doing the best I can for my child and for myself." "I am a woman, separate from my children, who is worthy of feeling contentment and inner peace." Feelings of guilt and worry lead to internal unrest—not peace.*

◆ Practice empathy, while teaching responsibility.

◆ Listen closely to your child's feelings and concerns. Take three deep breaths before responding. Ask yourself if what you are going to say will empower him to deal with his own issue, or if it will give him the message that he is unable to handle it and therefore you should handle it for him. Your job here is to keep the issue *his* and support him through it, while separately managing your own feelings and thoughts.

◆ Model emotional intelligence—the capacity to be aware of, control, and express one's emotions, and to handle interpersonal relationships judiciously and empathetically—by monitoring your own emotions when dealing with your child's issue, and by allowing yourself to step back and gain some clarity (or calm yourself down) when your emotions run high.

◆ Children learn how to handle and express their emotions by watching their parents. Be aware of how you handle yourself during times of elation, stress, sadness, and disappointment, and understand that your children will model this. If you want them to learn emotional intelligence, make sure that you are keeping yours in check by talking to other adults about your issues and by being mindful about what and how you share with your children.

◆ Let go. Connect with your faith and allow yourself to surrender to your higher power. Trust that if you *do* let go and establish and maintain healthy boundaries, your children will be okay, and so will you. I have been relieved to connect more deeply with my Jewish faith as a mother because it allows me to trust in G-d, which takes away some of the insane amounts of pressure I put on myself.

◆ Continually remind yourself of your innermost passions, and keep a pulse on your hopes, dreams, and desires (list them). Try to live them out in some measure as often as you can while your children are living with you.

SECURE YOUR IDENTITY AND ALLOW VULNERABILITY

Another important aspect of creating healthy emotional boundaries is making sure to secure your own identity while mothering your children, and allowing your children to see you for who you are. Know who you are, what you like, what you believe in, and what your values are, so that your self-esteem remains strong when life with children will challenge you to the core.

Along with maintaining a strong sense of self, both you and your children should also understand that you won't always know what to do or how to handle things that come your way. While you want your children to be able to draw strength from you so that you can be a role model to them as they develop their own sense of identity and security, it is also okay for you to admit to them that you have no clue what you are doing sometimes, and that you are just doing the best you can with who you are as a person and as a mother.

For me, because of my difficult and painful early years and the trauma I experienced as a teen, I have needed to do a great deal of work on strengthening my identity. Therapy, yoga, hypnosis, and meditation have all helped me with this, but I think part of my struggle with boundaries has much to do with not being as solidly grounded within myself as I would like to be, so I am more prone to take on my children's stuff to fill up some of the emptiness and uncertainty within myself. I know this about myself, and yet I still struggle.

I noticed this come out especially when my oldest daughter approached seventeen years old, the age I was when I got sick. I started to hover over her with a fervor that was almost obsessive. I worried about her nonstop and asked her far too many questions about every aspect of her life. When she called me out on it, I found myself opening up to her about how my battle with an eating disorder had left scars in the form of overprotectiveness, and how I wanted her never to experience the pain that I had experienced at her age. The more we talked about it, the more I felt the understanding between us grow, which gave me the strength to give her the space she needed to flourish on her own. I was able to practice better self-care by not feeling as if I needed to be as involved in her life, and I released myself from some of the unfounded worry I carried around.

The earlier you learn to define and honor your physical and emotional boundaries, the better able you will be to secure your identity, and the better off you'll be in the long run. Just as it happened with me, your own children will grow up, leave your nest, and carry on with their lives. When they are out from under your wing and are trying to establish themselves as contributing members of society (we hope!), you will be forced to do some re-establishing of yourself. You may ask yourself questions about who you are and what you like, need, and want, as your children's school, activities, or desires will no longer influence or direct your answers as much.

When my oldest daughter left for college, I truly felt like someone had sawed off one of my limbs; this year, 2015, my other son heads off to school, and I feel the same uncomfortable sensation of having a piece of my heart scooped out from my body. Thankfully, during my years of parenting I did not give up my passion for writing or for teaching fitness. I tried my best at maintaining relationships with good friends and a strong relationship with my husband. And, of course, I have another five and eight years, respectively, before my younger two exit the nest—or at least that is the plan. I do not wish to rush or slow down the remaining time I have with children in my house. I simply want to be more present during this time. The initial distress of having kids leave for college was a wake-up call about how fleeting the time that we have with our children is, and how it is so important for moms not only to cherish that time, but to continue to cultivate their own identities and nurture their other relationships.

CHAPTER 8:

Self-Care Solution #6—Nurture Your Partnership

"When you have a baby, you set off an explosion in your marriage, and when the dust settles, your marriage is different from what it was."

—*Nora Ephron*, Heartburn

My husband and I were married on a ridiculously cold, snowy day in November 1992 in St. Paul, Minnesota. While we were blissfully in love, we both realized very early on in our marriage that our journey together would be fiery—as in both passionate and loving, and testy and argumentative. It is who we are as individuals, as a couple and, as much as I hate to admit it, sometimes as parents as well. We are both strong willed, type A, and perfectionistic, and we have high expectations of ourselves and others.

Over the twenty-four years we have spent together as of the writing of this book—twenty-two of them as husband and wife, and twenty of them as parents—we have experienced some incredible highs and some devastating lows, and lots of in-betweens. The highs have included the birth of each one of our four children, the laughter we share, the fun we have as often as possible, and quite simply the deep love, care, and respect we have for one another.

And then, of course, there are the lows. All couples endure them, and about half make it through. There are the lows that can be categorized as nagging annoyances, like how he hates the way I load the dishwasher or how my blood boils over when he leaves dirty dishes in the sink. Sometimes seemingly trivial irritations can have deeper roots and can pile up over time. If couples do not take the necessary time and energy to work through issues as they come up, anger and resentment can grow past the point of no return. In addition to small issues becoming big issues, there are also times when couples bump up against real obstacles that can seem insurmountable. Some of the most difficult times in my marriage occurred when my husband and I realized that we had opposing views on parenting, family, friends, money, and intimacy. These were times when I would have welcomed a squabble over dishes left in the sink. These were times when our voices would drown each other out, when neither of us felt like we were being heard, respected, or even loved. Maybe we admitted this and maybe we didn't, but I know there were times when we were both unhappy and wondered if we would be happier without the other, and truly questioned if the grass might be greener elsewhere.

This is where the concept of self-care comes into play once again. Just as it is a choice to take care of yourself physically and emotionally, it is a choice to take care of yourself relationally. Your relationship with your partner is not one to be taken for granted, or neglected. As with all aspects of self-care, relational self-care is about intentionally treating your relationship with respect, love, care, attention, loyalty, and gratitude. It is about developing and maintaining healthy habits around communications and intimacy, and being aware when the relationship habits you and your partner have developed are no longer working and need to be adjusted. According to wife and husband Ashley Davis Bush and Daniel Arthur Bush, coauthors of 75 *Habits For a Happy Marriage—Marriage Advice to Recharge and Reconnect Every Day*, "The key to a great marriage is the quality of the habits you share together. Healthy, positive habits create an extraordinarily happy marriage. Negative habits create chronic dissatisfaction."

My husband and I have certainly had times when our relationship habits became infested with too much negativity and were steering us in a direction where neither of us were very satisfied. During a particularly rough spot, we received a pivotal piece of advice from a therapist that I think about almost daily: *Every single day is a choice to stay married. On any given day, at any given moment, either partner can walk out the door.*

The statement seems obvious and elementary, but what it said to me in such a loud and clear way is that, just as it is a choice to care for myself physically, emotionally, mentally, and spiritually, I need to be intentional and mindful about caring for my relationship with my partner. There is no question that marriage is tricky. You have two individuals who are each changing and evolving in their own ways, and simultaneously trying to evolve as a couple. Throw a few kids into the mix, and it can become very complicated. It is essential that neither you nor your partner takes the relationship for granted, and the key to preventing this is to practice relational self-care by actively infusing your relationship with heavy doses of respect, love, loyalty, and connection.

I have certainly seen all sorts of messy dynamics over the years. I know people who are counting the days until their kids are out of the house so they can leave their spouse, women and men who have had affairs, some of whom have stayed with their spouses and others who have left, and friends who truly dislike their spouse but stay because they are afraid to leave—afraid of the repercussions from their spouse, afraid for the kids, afraid of the financial ramifications, and afraid to be alone. I also know plenty of women who are truly happy in their relationship, and continue to be in love with their spouse or partner. Most moms, myself included, have run the full gamut of those feelings.

So, as I combine the analysis of my own marriage with three years of poring through hundreds of interviews with moms, I have come to my own conclusions about how to make your partnership successful and happy, and they center around these two key elements.

The first and most essential component to keeping your relationship strong is: You have to *want* it to work, and *believe* that it *can* work.

It sounds very simple, but sometimes it does come down to this. You have to have the will to make it work, and you have to understand that it is not easy, that you most likely will go through times when you will want to throw in the towel. But like anything, the more you work at it, the better it is going to be, and the more you will get out of it. Of course, the ideal scenario is that both partners are on the same page with this desire and commitment, and that both are willing to muddle through the inevitable rough spots that every couple experiences. But sometimes—probably more often than not—one person is the driving force that keeps the relationship on track. You may need to be the one who takes the reins of your struggling relationship—the one who plots out the date nights, makes the appointment with a therapist, initiates the difficult conversations. And hopefully your partner joins you on your journey to make things better.

The second component to a strong relationship is that it is imperative that you think of your partner not only as someone who makes you happy (or whom you expect to make you happy), but as someone whom you truly want to make happy. When most couples fall in love, each person is filled with a wonderful euphoria as they claim with certainty, "This woman/man makes me so happy." But ultimately, as time goes on, the individual realizes that the other person can't or won't always make them happy. Instead of becoming resentful and developing a "What has he done for me lately?" or "He doesn't understand me and never will" attitude, the healthy response—and one that works to foster a more meaningful and authentic partnership—is not to focus on what you are not getting, but to look at yourself and make sure you are sharing your whole heart with him so that he feels loved, valued, and connected to you. It is also important to ask yourself how honest you are being with your partner about your own needs, sensitivities, triggers, and insecurities, so that instead of assuming that your partner "should just know" certain things about you, you allow yourself to share these things with him. Allowing yourself to be vulnerable gives your partner a better chance at being able to show a deeper level of compassion and care (if they don't, this could be a problem). And possibly, with good communication on both sides of the relationship, your partner will also expose deeper layers of himself or herself so that you can be more aware and sensitive to his or her needs. Self-care in a relationship requires both partners to be intentional about caring for themselves and each other emotionally, physically, and mentally. A fulfilling and happy relationship happens when both partners feel valued and respected, and care deeply about their own happiness *and* the happiness of their partner.

Sometimes, however, a relationship may get so far off track that any of your efforts to pull the two of you back together feel futile. If your spouse is completely resistant to compromise or change and makes statements like "It's all your fault that you are not happy," or "If you don't like me the way I am then that's your problem," then it may be time for you to reevaluate. It does take the effort of both partners to make your relationship strong and healthy, and even though you may try your hardest to salvage your marriage and keep your family together, you cannot do all the work for both of you. And you certainly are not doing yourself or your kids any favors by staying in a miserable relationship. Sometimes couples really do grow apart. They reach uncomfortable places of boredom or monotony, or endure incessant, high levels of frustration in their relationship. Sometimes couples do not love or even like each other any more, and truly cannot find any joy in the relationship.

Experiencing certain amounts of any one of these feelings is virtually inevitable for couples at various points in their relationships. I am in the throes of perimenopause, and my husband just turned fifty and joined a band; it has taken a tremendous amount of patience, love, loyalty, and communication to get through some of these major life transitions. I am grateful that David and I have been practicing relational self-care for most of our marriage because it makes getting through the tough spots a little bit easier. If the pattern has been established to deal with relationship issues head-on, instead of continually sweeping them under the rug, it gives couples a fighting chance to stay together.

If, however, you are in a physically, mentally, or verbally abusive relationship, you must be prepared to leave if your or your children's safety is in jeopardy or if your partner is unwilling to get change or get help. But keep in mind that, whatever you do in regards to your relationship, it is imperative that you take care of yourself within your relationship, and to remember that your relationship is a model for your children. Your kids are all eyes and ears; they observe and learn from your partnership, even if you don't want them to. It is important for all concerned that your relationship be a strong model, and if it is not, that you work on a solution that makes sense for you and your family.

Just as you need to prioritize taking care of yourself while taking care of your family, you also need to carve out time to connect with your partner. The following mothers reveal the importance of nurturing their relationship with their spouse or partner as a component of their self-care prescription throughout their parenting journey.

> *In all honesty, the births of our children account for three of the four toughest times in our marriage. When you add a human being to a relationship, life and the relationship are forever changed. You either learn to acclimate and adjust or your relationship will wither. We also had to learn how to still be ourselves, as well as husband and wife before we were mom and dad. We had to learn that it's not selfish to put our needs ahead of our kids' wants.*
>
> —*MOTHER OF THREE CHILDREN,*
> *ages fifteen, twelve, and nine*

> *Any problems you might have with your spouse are magnified one hundred percent with children, and new issues are likely to arise. One friend mentioned that they*

were madly in love and could not have been happier, until they had children. Suddenly, they were talking about divorce. There is no running from yourself or each other. If you do, everyone will suffer. Be prepared to grow and change, otherwise things will more likely get worse and worse.

—*MOTHER OF TWO CHILDREN,*
age twelve (twins)

Nothing can substitute for a strong marriage. Having kids is hard work and it does take away from your energy and marriage, no matter how much you want kids. To parent well, you need to have a strong bond. Kids benefit from a united set of parents in so many ways.

—*MOTHER OF A FOUR-YEAR-OLD*

Try to remember that parenting is important and we usually put our children first but your relationship [with your partner] is so important. It really helps for children to see their parents have a healthy relationship. If possible, take time for each other, and sometimes have the kids be second—not always the center of attention.

—*MOTHER OF TWO CHILDREN,*
ages twenty-six and twenty-three

MAINTAIN A STRONG CONNECTION WITH YOUR PARTNER

Maintaining your connection as a couple as you raise your family is something that needs continual attention and effort. It is essential not to take your relationship with your partner for granted. Furthermore, do not assume that your children will be the glue that holds you together. In fact, having a child can often add additional strain to your relationship. So, just as you nurture your children, it is essential to nurture your relationship. Make sure you have open and supportive communication, a healthy sex life and physical intimacy (although it will not be quite the same as it was), and the time to do things together that you both enjoy.

"Try to treat your relationship with your partner as the one that's most important in your life—even more than the one with your children—and the whole family will benefit from it," says John Rosemond, family psychologist and author of *John Rosemond's New Parent Power*.[37] Of course this doesn't mean that parents should forget about their kids' needs, and it is natural for there to be some relationship neglect during the first years of a child's life. But couples can do small things that will convey to each other, and to the kids, how much they value their relationship. Journalist Teri Cettina encourages the practice of "creating warm welcomes." "Sure, you hug your kids and pet your dog every day," she writes. "But do you greet your husband with the same enthusiasm? Once in a while, kiss and hug as if one of you is going away and you aren't going to see each other for a week. Let the kids giggle: This kind of affection reassures them that you're close to each other, as well as to them."[38]

Another key component of continually maintaining the connection in your relationship is to work on effectively communicating with your partner. Communication also includes listening, really listening, to your partner even when you don't agree with him or her. All of my research, interviews, and personal experience point to the fact that open, honest, constructive, respectful communication is the key to a successful partnership. It is not the only component, but without this piece, all the other pieces become more fragile and can easily break. As individuals grow and change throughout their lives, communication is the way in which couples can understand and support one another and the partnership.

The most difficult times in my marriage have been when my husband and I were "two ships passing in the night," when he was traveling and busy with work and I was home with small kids. We had little time or energy to talk about issues as they would arise, so resentments would build up, needs would go unmet, and then things would boil over between us. It took us a long time to develop good strategies for managing conflict, and I can tell you with certainty that avoidance is not an effective tool for a healthy partnership. Figuring out how to "fight" is an essential part of a successful relationship and is also important for you and your partner to model for your children. Remember to hear each other out, and that if one person "wins" a fight, you both lose. A harmonious relationship involves a tremendous amount of compromise. It requires being able to assert your feelings, thoughts, and opinions, while respecting your partner's as well. As you work to practice self-care within your relationship by using effective communications strategies, make sure to avoid making assumptions like:

- He *must* understand how I am feeling. He should "just know," so I don't need to explain myself to him.
- If he loved me, he would understand how I am feeling.
- I know what he wants and what he needs; I don't really need to ask him.

ESSENTIAL TIPS FOR EFFECTIVE COMMUNICATION AND STRENGTHENING YOUR BOND WITH YOUR PARTNER

- It's never too early to begin discussing parenting styles and discipline strategies with your spouse. In fact, ideally this is something you will do even before you agree to get married. But if you haven't already begun doing this, now is the time to ask your partner hypothetical questions like: "What would you do if you caught our teenager drinking?" and "What if you think your daughter's best friend is a bad influence?" Issues like these may seem far off if you have young children, but it is very helpful to find out if you are on the same page with your partner well before you are in crisis. If you realize that you are not on the same page, you will have time to find common ground.

- Always back each other up when dealing with kids' issues, unless you feel that your partner has crossed the line and is being abusive.
- Share responsibilities: household, kids, finances, scheduling. Divide and conquer through discussions.
- Talk about money, one of the biggest stressors in a marriage. Discuss finances early on in your relationship and continue discussions regularly. Consider bringing in or hiring a third party to help you manage your finances. Be honest with each other about your spending and your wish lists. Talk about how much money it costs to raise kids (for a child born in 2013, approximately $300,000 over eighteen years),[39] and whether you plan to pay for some or all of their college. Discuss how you are going to save for your retirement.
- Understand that marriage is challenging and that it is not "supposed" to be easy or fun all the time. Demonstrate patience and belief in yourself and in each other.
- Set aside weekly time for just the two of you. Be deliberate about this, even if it is just one night a week after the kids go to sleep, when you can just focus on being together, talking, and connecting without distractions.
- When you are together, make sure that the conversation goes beyond kid-related issues.
- Plan fun things to do together and incorporate laughter into your relationship as often as possible. Go dancing or bowling, see funny movies or plays, watch funny TV shows together, or spend time with friends whom you both enjoy.
- What are the elements in your relationship with your

partner that are the most satisfying for you?

- ◆ What are the biggest sticking points in your relationship?
- ◆ Do you address these issues with your partner? How?
- ◆ How do you deal with conflict? How does your partner? Talk about conflict resolution when you are not in the middle of a conflict.
- ◆ Do you feel like you get most of your needs met in the relationship? Do you feel that you are able to meet most of your partner's needs? If either or both of these answers are no, do you talk about your unmet needs with your partner? Are you receptive to your partner sharing his or her unmet needs?
- ◆ How often do you have meaningful conversations with your partner? How often would you like to?
- ◆ How often do you and your partner spend time alone? How often would you like to?
- ◆ Are you in love with your partner?
  - *If so, what are the things that you love about your partner?*
  - *If not, do you remember falling out of love with your partner and can you identify what it would take to reignite the love?*
- ◆ Can you visualize a "better," healthier relationship with your partner?
  - *What does it look and feel like?*
  - *What needs to change in order for you to make this vision a reality?*

MAINTAINING YOUR SENSE OF SELF IN THE RELATIONSHIP

As important as it is to join your partner in the process of raising your children, one of the best ways to do this—which so many moms do not understand from the get-go—is to take care of yourself. The most successful relationships I have seen throughout my life and throughout my interviews are those in which both partners are securely invested in taking good care of their own happiness and well-being, as well as showing great care and concern for their partner's happiness and well-being. Each partner has a high level of self-respect as well as a strong respect for his or her partner.

This is the model which I strive for with my husband, and what I have learned is that while there is no way any couple will always be perfectly in sync, the most important component of a strong, healthy, balanced partnership is a strong, healthy, balanced *you*. And in order to be so, you need to practice what we've discussed in the first five chapters of this book, so that you can feel good about who you are and what you contribute to your partner and the relationship, and be clear on what you need from your partner. Questions to consider include:

- How do you take care of yourself in your relationship with your partner?
- Do you ever feel as if you are more concerned about pleasing your partner than you are about advocating for your own happiness?
- Do you feel that you are able to assert yourself with your spouse?
- Do you feel like you are an "equal" partner in the relationship (emotionally, financially)?
- What are your needs in your relationship? Are you able to effectively communicate them with your partner?
- Do you feel safe in your relationship? Emotionally, mentally, physically?
- Do you feel that your partner treats you with love, honor, and respect?

If there are any red flags that come up for you as you explore the above questions, make sure that you talk to your partner or to a friend about any issues you may be having. Just as many women "lose themselves" when they become mothers, women and mothers also claim to lose their sense of self when they become the "pleaser" in their relationship with their spouse. And if at any time you do not feel safe with your partner, please call for help immediately.

CO-PARENTING: MAINTAINING
A UNITED FRONT

It is only a matter of time before parents realize that you can run but you can't hide. Children see right through you. They study you and quickly learn where your hot buttons are; they see your issues, your dysfunction, and your differences in opinions and parenting styles. They are usually able to find the weak link in your relationship and know how and when to pounce in an effort to move their own agenda forward.

I remember a monster fight my husband and I got into when my oldest daughter was maybe four. We were on our way up to a cousin's cabin for the July Fourth weekend and I started talking about how fun it would be for our daughter to go inner-tubing. My husband went a little crazy. He said, "She is *not* going inner-tubing! She is four years old! That is way too dangerous!" I said, "Well, I think my dad said he would take her." He said, "No way! That is crazy. She is not doing that! Why do you make those kinds of decisions without consulting me?!" The outcome was that my husband and I did not speak for the whole day at the cabin, and I'm pretty sure that my dad did end up taking my daughter on the tube and she survived. And my husband and I talked about the fact that he is more of the stereotypical "Jewish mother" parent, while I am a little less rigid but sometimes inconsistent.

Fast-forward ten years to a scene at our dinner table, where the same daughter, now fourteen, started talking about how excited she was to go to a Taylor Swift concert. My husband scrunched up his brow and began asking her a series of questions that included: "Who is taking you? Is this person staying at the concert with you? How are you getting home?" He did not like the answers, so he simply stated, "You are not going."

Whoa! Brace for impact! My daughter was begging me through her sobs to talk some sense into Dad. My husband was voicing his disappointment to me about how I don't consult with him when making decisions. I was defending myself and reminding him that he had just been out of the country on a weeklong business trip, and I had had to hold down the fort and make all sorts of decisions on my own that included this one, which I still believed was a fine decision . . . and our three other children were on the edge of their seats.

The tubing issue, the Taylor Swift concert (which she did end up going to, chaperoned)—well, those were just a few that caused some tumult. Others were: Can she go to the party at a friend's house (whom you have never heard of and whose parents you certainly don't know)? Can he go to the homecoming after-party? Can you host the prom after-party? These parenting decisions can cause a tremendous amount of stress. Each parent brings so much to the table when making these types of decisions, and kids are quick to figure out how to work the system. It can be helpful for couples to talk about decision making very early on: How were decisions made in your house growing up? Was one parent the softy who always—with enough coaxing—gave in, and the other the "no budging" parent?

One mother of six talked about the challenges of keeping her kids on a "narrow road" and how to manage this when she and her husband have different parenting styles, explaining, "My husband is a cement barricade and I am more of a bumper."

The key to guiding your children and staying aligned with your partner is to keep communicating. You will most definitely not agree on every aspect of raising your children, but as you will hear from many mothers, showing respect for one another and backing each other up on issues is an essential piece of taking care of your relationship while taking care of your children. The relationship between the parents is the foundation upon which the family system is built. The system will function much more effectively if the foundation is solid. If your relationship is not solid and if your united front is not clearly communicated—

particularly when dealing with teens—further deterioration is often the result, and the rift can be detrimental to the children.

I have known mothers and wives who are so unhappy with their husbands that they share their disappointments and frustrations with their kids, effectively 'ganging up' on Dad. Or it might be the other way around, where Dad sends a message to the children that Mom is 'completely out to lunch' and 'doesn't have a clue.' How can this work? It can't. The gang-up strategy is toxic to every relationship—parent-to-parent and parent-to-child. Plain and simple, don't do it. It is okay for your kids to see you and your partner not agreeing on every issue; in fact, it is essential. They need to learn conflict resolution. They need to see you model healthy assertive behavior, to hear you express an opinion and explain your point of view.

However, it is not okay to involve your kids in a conflict with your partner or show disrespect for your partner in front of them. A study in the April 2009 *Journal of Family Psychology* suggests that kids who get pulled into their parents' conflicts are at a higher risk for developing symptoms of depression and anxiety.[40]

Communication gaps, inconsistencies in parenting styles, and even subtle differences in where to draw the line with your children can affect your relationship with your partner. The most important lesson I have learned through years of trial and error (and some World War III–level blowouts) is that when you realize you have hit a roadblock with your partner, and that the question your child needs an answer to *right now* cannot be answered that instant, it is just fine to tell her that you and your partner need to discuss the issue in private and that you will get back to her. For many couples this seems elementary, but it can get tricky, particularly when the parent who makes most of the small, day-to-day decisions makes a unilateral decision on something larger—like the concert—with which the other vehemently disagrees. This can be frustrating for both parents. Neither one is right or wrong; they simply have very different opinions about the issue. Teens will pick up on this and try to weigh in, further complicating matters. The most detrimental thing a couple can do is to get into a power struggle and start judging one another for their respective opinions.

Differences in the ways that each partner was parented often come into play as they reach unknown territory with their children. Most parents fall back on their own experience, and either want to do things completely differently than what their parents did, or stick with what they know: "I was going to concerts with my friends, without parent chaperones, at age fourteen and I turned out okay," I reminded my husband during our Taylor Swift disagreement. "Well, I wasn't," he snapped. "My parents would never have let me."

Once again, no one is right or wrong, but together you need to find a common ground, along the lines of: "Okay, we both want her to have fun and enjoy the concert of one of her favorite musicians, but we want her to be safe. How can we make that happen?" It is essential for parents to remain true to their individual values as well as to each other. When kids figure out that Mom is the yea-sayer and Dad is the nay-sayer, you know whom they are going to go to when they want something. This good-cop/bad-cop scenario is both divisive and destructive to the family system. Partners must work together to guide their children; when they do not agree on an issue, the prudent course is to talk through the issue behind closed doors and reach a consensus in order to present a united front.

The following moms talk about how they make co-parenting work:

> *Work together and never undermine your spouse's parenting methods! Both you and your hubby make the rules and you both need to make sure the children follow them. Always back up your spouse. If you don't agree with the other's methods, talk about it away from the children and come up with something you both will agree on.*
>
> —*MOTHER OF TWO CHILDREN, did not provide ages*

Fight the problem, not each other. It's something that my husband's grandparents started and it has been a family tradition since then.

—MOTHER OF FOUR CHILDREN,
*ages fifteen, twelve, eight, and two,
and three stepchildren*

Number one is to back each other up when one of you disciplines the children. No matter if you feel that your spouse has done it the wrong way, you can talk about it later and learn from that. If you start to tell your significant other that he's parenting your child wrong in front of [the child], eventually your children start to see one of you as insignificant. ([Assuming] of course, your spouse is not physically abusing the kids.)

—MOTHER OF THREE CHILDREN,
ages eight, six, and three

LET'S TALK ABOUT SEX

When I surveyed mothers about the biggest stressor in their relationship with their partner, not surprisingly, fifty-three percent of respondents said it was money. What did surprise me, however, was that sex, or lack thereof, came in a close second (with children third, managing priorities fourth, and work fifth). There is no question that the financial, physical, and emotional responsibilities of caring for a family can create a disconnect for couples. And sex and intimacy are bound to take a hit. Many of the divorced moms I surveyed claimed that their partner's infidelity was the cause of their divorce. Whether or not we want to admit it, sex is important.

The time and energy that previously was reserved for couple time becomes more limited and is often sacrificed altogether in service to kid-related needs or wants. But these interviews, and my own personal experience, point to the fact that this ultimately does not make us happy and that we do crave intimacy with our partners. At the very least, we realize that there is a problem when we do not experience intimacy with our partners on a regular basis. Typically, men are known to focus more on the physical act of sex and women on the relational intimacy, which involves:

◆ Meaningful conversations
◆ Hand-holding
◆ Spending one-on-one time together without distractions
◆ Subtle words or actions that indicate that you are loved and cherished by your partner

However, plenty of women crave sex as well, just as many men yearn for intimacy. The following mothers share their feelings about the levels of intimacy in their relationships, and the difficulties parents face as they try to find time for intimacy within their hectic and busy lives as parents.

> *We have a phenomenal partnership; it's the level of intimacy that's missing for us. We share the same values, the same life vision, the same priorities (overall) regarding the children and their education and activities. The issues we have are with my husband not being able to meet me halfway. He struggles with listening and although he is an excellent talker, not such a great listener. He's working on it though!*
>
> —MOTHER OF TWO CHILDREN, ages seven and five

> *[I try to make time for] intimacy with my hubby and not always sex either, just REALLY knowing that he is there for me to let it out all on even if I'm frantic when it all comes out.*
>
> —MOTHER OF A TWO-YEAR-OLD

*Whenever we do get the chance to go out alone, we
really do have fun—and I want to hold hands and I do
see us growing old together. Although alone times are
few and far between, those feelings I feel when we are
alone are the 'light at the end of the tunnel' when we're
not connecting or when life seems so chaotic.*

—MOTHER OF TWO CHILDREN,
ages four and two

If sex and intimacy are issues for half of all couples I surveyed, I would not be afraid to go out on a limb and conclude that this speaks to the population in general. The failure to nurture the relationship with your partner inevitably leads to dissatisfaction for both partners, which can lead to infidelity and/or the complete demise of the partnership.

The question becomes, what can mothers do to try to make things more satisfying for themselves and for their partners? There is no question that there needs to be two willing parties to keep a partnership healthy and strong, but sometimes one person needs to take the lead on reading the barometric pressure of the relationship.

In the fall of 2014, an Orthodox rabbi came to our home to speak to us about our connection to Judaism, among many other things. Neither my husband nor I is an Orthodox Jew, but we find this particular rabbi and his teachings extremely thought-provoking, and study with him every other month. We landed on the topic of relationships and marriage, and he explained to my husband, our teenage son, and me how in the Orthodox community, a boy/man does not ever touch another girl/woman, other than his mother and/or sisters, until he is married, and at that point, his wife is the only woman he can touch (he can still hug his mother and sisters). The same goes for girls/women. So, when an Orthodox man and woman get married, they have never hugged, held hands, or touched in any way, let alone had sex.

"So how do you know when you meet the girl that you want

to marry?" my son asked curiously.

"You know because you know her intimately. You spend hours and hours getting to know the person she is, you are aware of her every mood; how she acts when she is happy, sad or upset; you find out who she is at the deepest level possible, and she gets to know you in the same way," explained the rabbi. And yet, this process does not involve any physical contact.

At this point, some moms who are reading this are standing up and cheering, "Yes! See, I told you sex is overrated!" But once an Orthodox Jewish couple is married, sex does become an integral part of their relationship (especially as it relates to procreation) and there are a lot of rituals around sex, which I will not examine for the purposes of this book. But the issues of sex *and* intimacy are both important, and for extraordinarily busy and overscheduled couples today, these issues must be discussed. Both partners need to be mindful and deliberate about making sure that sex and intimacy remain a priority.

When I asked the women who listed sex as one of the main stressors in their relationship what they were doing to deal with this issue, I could almost feel them shaking their bowed heads. Many women said something along the lines of "nothing" or "ignoring it." One mother of a fifteen-year-old, who has been married eighteen years, responded, "Drink and smoke." And for some mothers, this issue was the straw that broke the relationship: "Got divorced." Other mothers reveal how they are struggling with this issue and how they deal with it:

> [I] whine, complain, get upset, which only makes it worse. It has become awkward and uncomfortable, like every time is the first time all over again. It doesn't feel like it comes naturally to either of us anymore.
> —MOTHER OF A TWO-YEAR-OLD

> It's more difficult to get the intimacy we both want. Also physically, in the time it takes my body to go back to normal after having a baby (about the time I start

getting a period again). I have very little sexual desire.

—*MOTHER OF TWO CHILDREN,*
ages two and one

At the end of the day, I've had enough physical contact,
between holding and nursing the baby all day, and
playing with my two-year-old. My poor husband is
lucky to get a hug and maybe a quick kiss from me
when he gets home. That's about the extent of affection
I have left after the kids have zapped out the rest!

—*MOTHER OF TWO CHILDREN,*
ages two and five months

[My spouse] thinks more sex would solve our problems.
I think if we could figure out how to manage priorities,
money and sex [issues] would solve themselves.

—*MOTHER OF TWO CHILDREN,*
ages two and six weeks

FIND INTIMACY AS A WAY
TO CONNECT WITH YOUR PARTNER

Now if I wanted to be really blunt, I could ask the question that most moms, at some or many points in their daily lives as mothers, want to scream from the rooftops: "What am I supposed to do about the fact that I feel exhausted, hormonal, crabby, underappreciated, and unsexy, and that I often crave time and space in which no one needs or demands anything from me physically, mentally, or emotionally? How am I supposed to get my sexy on when I barely have the time or energy to take a shower when I am home with my young kids all day?"

And this is only the tip of the iceberg for many moms in terms of why sex can be so difficult when they become mothers. Maybe you've let yourself go physically, or your partner has, and you don't feel attractive or feel attracted to your partner anymore. Maybe hormones and exhaustion truly have numbed your sex drive. How do you keep the connection strong and the spark alive in your relationship when the demands of parenting are so high and there are so many variables that come into play?

So often, the sex issue is one that commands so much attention for couples because it is tangible and measurable. The amount of sex a couple is having or not having can certainly be the flashing red light that illuminates a disconnect, but generally speaking, while sex is certainly an important component, the overall health of the relationship is dependent on a combination of many more factors. A healthy relationship starts with and is nurtured by a strong emotional connection, and quite often, the sex is an extension of that closeness and intimacy. In other words, working on the root causes of a couple's lack of intimacy and sex, instead of just focusing on how much or how little sex you are having, is often a more healthy and productive approach to bringing a couple closer together.

According to Barton Goldsmith, Ph.D., author of *Emotional Fitness for Intimacy*:

> *Intimacy doesn't mean having a sex life that rivals 50 Shades of Gray. Of course, true intimacy is much sweeter that that. It is an exchange of tender energy between two people who love each other deeply. The intimacy that you exchange with a loving partner can turn bad days into good ones and make your troubles seem much smaller. Without it, your ability to take on the world can be greatly compromised.*
>
> *The most important intimate moments are those that happen outside of the bedroom. Reaching your arms around your partner's waist and giving a squeeze when he or she is working away in the kitchen or around the house is very endearing. Holding hands while you are walking into a store or going out for a stroll together in the park is a bonding experience. There are countless ways to be intimate, and most of them aren't sexual.*[41]

ESSENTIAL TOOLS FOR SEX AND INTIMACY:

◆ Be mindful of how sex, intimacy, and feeling connected are all essential components of a healthy relationship.

◆ Pay attention to your partner every single day. Be generous about showing him or her your love.

◆ Be mindful of how you greet your partner. Do you smile, hug, or kiss when you see him or her?

◆ Be aware of how you talk to your partner. Pay attention to your tone. Do you speak in a loving, caring voice, like you would speak to a really close friend?

◆ Do you say "I love you" regularly? Is it just a habit, or do you allow yourself to actually feel it when you say it and when you hear it from your partner?

◆ Notice the ways you show affection toward your partner. Do you ever hold hands or walk arm in arm?

◆ Make spending time with your partner a clear priority and be proactive about making it happen. Book a babysitter or send kids to grandma's. Make a dinner reservation or plan to stay in when the kids are out of the house. Let your partner know that you look forward to your time alone with him or her.

◆ List specific things you do or say every day that demonstrate your love for your partner.

◆ Are you open and receptive to the gestures your partner makes toward you that demonstrate his or her love?

◆ On a scale of one to ten, how would you rate your sex drive? How would you rate your partner's?

◆ Do you and your partner agree on how often you would like to be or "should" be having sex? If not, how far apart are you?

◆ Talk about sex with your partner: communicate regularly about your needs, wants and desires (and lack thereof).

- Make plans for intimacy. As busy as life gets, sometimes couples need to carve out time and plan for sex. Spontaneity may not be a viable option at this stage of life, although you can certainly look for such opportunities.
- Are you still attracted to your partner?
- Do you feel that your partner is attracted to you?
- If the answer to the last two questions was no, what are you going to do about this serious issue? Can you have this conversation with your partner in a constructive way?
- Look for ways to keep the love and the spark alive: send (or even text) love notes, light candles in your bedroom or bathroom and run a bath after your kids go to bed at night, hold hands, and hug and kiss often—and make sure your kids see these gestures of love and care (remember, you are modeling what a relationship looks and feels like).
- When you know you have time alone or a date night with your husband, make an attempt to practice extra self-care that day (maybe take a nap) so you will have enough energy to focus on the two of you, and so you are not falling asleep as your waiter is bringing dessert.
- If this is an area of struggle for you and your partner, make sure to talk about it. If talking does not work to make things better, you may need to seek professional help. Once again, you are making an investment in your relationship. Reminder: this investment is much cheaper and less time-consuming than divorce!
- Practice ongoing self-care. Exercising, eating well, and taking time to ground yourself provides you with more energy and helps you feel better about yourself in general, which spills over to how you see yourself as a partner and a lover. Self-care also provides you

with the "fuel" that you need to be better able to be more loving and giving to your partner.

KEYS TO A STRONG PARTNERSHIP

Just as you approach anything in your life that is important to you—like your job, or your parenting—your relationship needs to be approached with a similar kind of commitment and high level of importance. If neglected, there is no question that it will go stale. The following mothers reveal their advice for keeping your partnership strong at every level:

> *Mommy does not equal sexy, so you need to get away and remember who you are as a whole person, what makes you feel good and excited about yourself and your spouse. My mom and dad had frequent date nights and I saw my mom looking sexy for my dad and I think that was a great example for me. I can be both, [mom and sexy wife], and it keeps me in tune with my husband. And we both understand that in this society, marriage does not necessarily mean forever. We have choices and we have to decide to stay together through the hard times. We have weathered some really tough times in our seven years together and have gotten stronger each time we've recommitted to one another.*
>
> —*MOTHER OF A TWO-YEAR-OLD*

> *[My husband] and I would try and make time with each other by having 'in home date nights' as soon as the kids went to bed. We would light a candle, drink some wine and watch a movie or listen to music together or just talk and catch up. It was also easy on the budget and we didn't have to get all dressed up, get a sitter, etc.*
>
> —*MOTHER OF TWO CHILDREN,*
> *ages fifteen and thirteen*

The best marital advice I can give is to make time for yourselves as a couple. When my first child was born, I was living in the suburbs of New York with no friends with kids. I was lonely, tired and bored being stuck at home with a newborn who cried a lot. I remember reading an advice column in a magazine for new moms. It stressed that no man wants to come home to a wife who hasn't gotten dressed and is covered in baby food. It also said not to say no to sex. It stressed that everyone is tired but that you can't let 'tired' ruin your relationship. I have followed those two bits of advice for 18 years. I have a good marriage. No matter how crappy my day was I made sure that I was showered and dressed by the time my husband came home from work even if it meant showering with one foot rocking my infant in his seat. We go out on regular date nights and I put a lot of effort into making sure that we have couple time. Every marriage has hills and valleys, and having kids is stressful. You need to talk to your husband, express your needs, and make time for each other.

*—MOTHER OF FOUR CHILDREN,
ages eighteen, sixteen, fourteen, and nine*

Some would argue that the above-quoted woman sounds a bit like a 1950s housewife. However, I know this woman, and she happens to be a very modern, accomplished, strong, independent woman who is a retired lawyer and a business owner. She and her husband have a wonderful, loving, "equal" relationship. The above-mentioned strategy works for them. My husband and I have been married for about the same amount of time and also have a very strong, loving relationship. While my husband might prefer me to be showered and dressed when we see each other at the end of the day, there are days when I am still in my yoga clothes when he walks in the door from work because I had a writing deadline or just because "I'm too tired," and this works just fine for us. The bottom line is that there is no magic, one-size-fits-all strategy for maintaining a healthy, happy, lasting relationship. You need to find what works for you as a couple and keep your communication open, and there is no getting around this: your relationship requires ongoing, intentional, and thoughtful care and attention. So for the health and well-being of yourself, your partner, your partnership, and your family, it is essential to remember that intentionally caring for your relationship is an integral part of your self-care solution.

CHAPTER 9:

Self-Care Solution #7 — Find Work-Life Balance

"It probably takes more endurance, more patience, more intelligence, more healthy emotion, to raise a decent, happy human being than to be an atomic physicist, a politician, or a psychiatrist."

—*Milton R. Sapirstein*, Emotional Security

No matter how you define work, there is no denying that once you hear your baby cry for the first time, you realize that it is your full-time job to ensure that her needs are met and that ultimately she attains the mental, physical, and emotional tools she will need to take care of herself. This massive responsibility will require you to *work* in ways you never have before, and your idea of what a *job* is will never be the same.

Whether they choose to stay home with their children, work part-time or full-time, work from home or outside of their home, many women struggle with the issue of whether or not to go back to work after they have children. For some women, the answer is readily available: they feel passionate about their work, or they need to provide for their family financially, or both. Some mothers, from a financial perspective, do have a choice whether or not to work for pay, but face their own challenges regarding finding purpose, fulfillment, and balance in their lives. The rewards and the challenges are very different for women who stay home full-time and women who work outside the home, but both situations are important, both deserve respect, and neither deserves judgment.

I had the privilege of hearing American author (*Alexander and the Terrible, Horrible, No Good, Very Bad Day*), newspaper journalist, and psychoanalysis researcher Judith Viorst speak at a Minneapolis Jewish Federation lunch in August 2013. The mother of three grown sons, a mother-in-law, and a grandmother, Viorst spoke about many different issues related to mothering and empowering women. She described what she calls a "marital democracy," the pattern that most married couples with children often fall into, wherein mom is the general manager of the family regardless of whether she is a stay-at-home mom or a working mom.

"She is the reminder of birthdays, important events," Viorst explained. "She has her antennae up to hurt feelings and knows when to intervene with our children, or not." And quite often, she added, "this system of having the wife/mother in charge of the family works well."

I don't think there is anything particularly sexist about this setup because moms usually just "get it." One of our many maternal powers is that it's in our DNA to be hyper-connected to all that needs to happen to ensure that our family functions somewhat properly—and we are usually more connected in this way than our male counterparts. However, what gets me sometimes, and seems to bother many other moms as well, is that the role of general manager of our family is often not held in as high esteem as, say, a general manager of a company is. I do understand that we are talking apples and oranges, but as women continue to fight their way to equal wages in the workplace and to shatter the glass ceiling that still exists, I see many bright, talented, creative moms (especially stay-at-home moms) struggling to feel confident in their roles. I certainly have been one of those moms at certain times in my life.

Before I became a mother and in my early stages of mothering, I subscribed to the idea that the provider of the family was the one who was "bringin' home the bacon." I had been vigorously attached to the feeling that unless I was working for a paycheck that I could contribute to the "pot," I was not fully pulling my weight. Well, I am here to tell you that, after nearly twenty-two years of marriage and twenty years of mothering (during some of which I have worked outside the home), I have proved myself dead *wrong*! Paycheck or no paycheck, I am a critical provider for my family. I provide clean laundry, clean dishes, healthy meals, a somewhat orderly, clean house (well, on most days), toilet paper in the bathrooms, school supplies, clothing and shoes that fit, and a stocked fridge (and freezer and pantry, because you never know when a half a dozen or more of the kids' friends are going to show up hungry). I am a cheerleader, avid spectator of all my kids' sports and performances, camp counselor, travel agent, entertainment coordinator, bookkeeper (which includes filling out countless forms for camp, school, Hebrew school, sports, lessons, etc.), payer of bills, coach, playmate, calendar keeper, and of course, a driver for the never-ending doctor, dentist, and orthodontist appointments, conferences, practices, games, meetings, haircuts, birthday parties, and playdates. I am an organizer, a tutor, a white-knuckled driving instructor, a makeshift nurse and doctor, a therapist, a manicurist, a hairstylist, a fashion consultant, a referee, a disciplinarian, and an engaged listener (to all the minutiae as well as the "big stuff" in my children's lives), *and* I take out the garbage.

But more than anything in the world, I am a giver of unconditional, unfaltering, unwavering *love* (even during the times when I feel so drained that it feels like there is nothing of me left to give). If that is not called providing, I don't know what is.

This is the basic job description for every mom today, give or take a few of these roles. And this is just the work she does in the house and with the kids. This list does not take into account the work she does outside the home, whether it is paid or volunteer. And how about the list that involves all we do for our partners, other family members, and friends? And after all of this, we still need to try to find time, sometimes only moments, for ourselves. Just taking a shower or going to the bathroom without a child coming in to talk to you or yelling for you from another room can be viewed as treasured time.

Helaine (a mother of two children, ages twenty and sixteen), who was involved with this book in its early stages, explains her situation:

> *Before I was married, one of my mother's friends asked me about what I would do about my work as a psychologist when I had children. I commented that I would get daycare for my kids. I loved my work and could never imagine not doing it. During one of my training experiences, a supervisor asked me the same question, and I had the same answer. She suggested to me that even if I did decide one day to stay home with my kids, that I should at least keep one foot in the door. It was her experience that women who stayed home full time lacked the confidence to get back into the work world once it came time.*
>
> *Here comes the irony: when my first child was born, I loved everything about being a parent. In my last month of my pregnancy I had stopped working, thinking that I would go back to work when my child was a few months old. As the months went by, the idea of going back to work slowly faded. Looking back, hindsight is not even twenty-twenty. I still do not know if I totally made the right decision. Yes, it would have definitely helped to have the extra income all of these years. But I was happy being home with my kids and helping out at their school. I would not trade my time with my children. But what I have sacrificed is a sense of success and a financial contribution to my family. At times, I feel that I have lost myself.*
>
> *There were days when I felt so out of the loop,*

wishing that I had I had taken the advice of my
supervisor and at least kept one foot in the door. With
that said, it worked for me—mostly.

What Helaine didn't realize is that she really did keep one foot in the door by staying active as a volunteer. Throughout the gestation of this book, Helaine rejoined the workforce. Her first job back was with a nonprofit agency, and then she came full circle and re-entered a private counseling practice working with children and families. She was able to get both of these jobs through contacts she made while volunteering. Helaine advises, "Do not underestimate volunteer work. I got my last job offer based on my volunteer work. I didn't even have to interview for the job! Your volunteer work can keep your résumé strong."

WORKING OUTSIDE THE HOME

Whether you are a single mom or part of a dual-income family, working part-time or full-time, most moms who work outside the home talk about feeling like they have to do it all. Once you overcome that obstacle of separating from your children—some moms actually welcome this separation, while others never really overcome their feelings of guilt—there are daily challenges. Mothers take multitasking to new levels: they simultaneously apply mascara and feed their baby a bottle; they fill cereal bowls and leave them out on the breakfast table the night before so they can get dressed for work as their children eat their Cap'n Crunch; they use their lunch break to run to the grocery store to get milk and peanut butter and store the milk in the staff room refrigerator, and pray that they won't forget it in there because the kids have not had milk in their cereal for three days. When Mom and Dad both work, questions like "Who stays home when the children are sick?" or "Who should stop at Target to pick up diapers on the way home from work?" or "Who should pick up Junior from day care and who should make dinner?" need to be negotiated on a regular basis. But interestingly enough, despite all the juggling that goes on every single day, most of the women

I surveyed and interviewed who work full- or part-time feel great fulfillment in their jobs—especially if they have some flexibility.

Needless to say, working moms must continually make tough and sometimes painful choices. In Letty Cottin Pogrebin's article "On Golda Meir" for the Jewish Women's Archive, Israeli prime minister Golda Meir describes a working woman's conundrum: "'I was always rushing from one place to another—to work, home, to a meeting, to take Menachem to a music lesson, to keep a doctor's appointment with Sarah, to shop, to cook, to work and back home again. And still, to this day,' [Meir] wrote at age seventy-seven, 'I am not sure that I didn't harm the children or neglect them.' At the same time, she acknowledged, 'There is a type of woman who cannot let her husband and children narrow her horizons.'"

My personal story does not parallel Meir's, but it does have to do with some of the same feelings of failure and the same admission that I was unable to do it all. I started working at the age of fifteen when my grandfather, who was in the fruit business, helped get me a job selling fruit at the farmer's market—start time was Saturday mornings at five a.m. So, at a young age, I realized how much I liked the feeling of fulfillment that I got from working, as well as how empowered I felt by earning my own money.

From that point on, I saw work as a necessity for me, something that gave me purpose and made me feel whole. I worked a variety of jobs throughout high school, and for two years during college, I worked three jobs at once. I worked at a local drugstore, at a summer day camp, at my dad's recycling center (hard hat and all!), at my college newspaper, as a ghostwriter for a book, and as an editorial assistant for a college professor who was writing a book; I waited tables, interned at a newspaper in Washington, DC and for a television news station in Minneapolis, taught various fitness classes, sold men's and women's clothing, wrote newsletters for several companies, and was an account executive at a public relations agency. I felt like I really understood the importance of working, of connecting with people, of being a team player.

But then something changed: I had a baby. I fooled myself into thinking that things would not change very much, and I was determined to keep my career thriving despite the beautiful, blue-eyed daughter of mine, with whom I fell madly in love the instant I saw her. I did, however, leave my full-time public relations job and found a half-time job writing for an educational consulting company. The job would provide me with much more flexibility and I could do much of my work at home but still have an office to go to. It was the perfect setup. And here is how perfect it was for me: barely two months into the job, something happened that I had never experienced before as an employee of dozens of companies for which I had worked over the past decade. I got "let go." My boss told me over the phone that "it just wasn't working out." In other words, *I* wasn't working out. And he was right. To this day, I cringe to think about the subpar work I turned in to him. And yet, at the time, it may have been the best I could do.

My hormones were raging, I wasn't sleeping, and I had a very tough time concentrating on any one thing for very long. When I was home, I was thinking I should be working, but I was too consumed and overwhelmed with all the unknowns of being a new mom and handling this dependent little being. When I was working, I was exhausted from not sleeping and busy worrying about my daughter, who I'd left with a babysitter I wasn't even sure if I liked. I was preoccupied with pumping breast milk, dealing with mastitis, and thinking about how much longer it would be until I got to see her—I could hardly focus on getting any real work done.

So, I left my "perfect" new job feeling embarrassed, ashamed, and like a complete failure. Millions of women have babies and go back to work because they have to, they want to, or both. What was wrong with me? Why couldn't I do it? I told myself at first that my failure came as a result of my not really liking the job, combined with the fact that, financially, I did not absolutely have to work at the time. But I think the bottom line, which I learned through trial and error, was that I really wanted to devote myself to being home with my baby girl, at least for a while.

As time went on and I emerged from my sleep-deprived fog, overcame the shame of my job termination and became a little more comfortable with being a new mom, I was able to think about working again. I eased myself back into some freelance writing work and began to teach fitness classes again. I was ready, and it felt good. I have never worked full-time since I became a mother, and I am truly in awe of those incredible women who do. I know how much time it takes to manage the basic mothering and household responsibilities, and I am amazed at how moms manage their full-time jobs, their children, their other relationships (often including the one with their partner) and their homes.

But the truth is that there is no perfect way to "do it all," and almost all mothers, at one point or another, feel as if something or someone is getting the short end of the stick. Children's musical artist Laurie Berkner wrote in the *Huffington Post*, "Every woman I know who has a job and is a parent has to deal every day with making enough time for both. I never really am able to do it. I just keep stealing from one part of my life to give to the other. (I figure by the time my daughter is in college, I'll be caught up.) Balancing it all is definitely one of the biggest sources of stress in my life, and one way I deal with stress is to write about it."

Life coach, author and yoga instructor, wife, and mother of two children Laura Erdman-Luntz, M.A., speaks to these challenges as well. During my interview with her, she revealed that her biggest challenge in her dual role is "mom guilt." She asked, "Do I spend enough time with my children? Do they know they are my priority even though I can't always choose them first? Will I feel I missed out on their youth when these precious years are gone?" In an effort to deal with these challenges, Laura revealed, "The most important thing for me is to make sure the time I do have with my children is quality time. I want to be fully present with them when we are together, as well as to be able to thoroughly enjoy them with my heart and soul."

However, Laura is equally committed to and clear on the value of her work. "I so enjoy my work and it is so deeply rewarding, I simply cannot imagine not doing it. Not only does that make me a happier, more satisfied mom, it also models to my children that you can live your dream. My children do not even have in their awareness that people could do work simply to pay the bills. They already assume their life's work is their life's purpose. I think that idea is one of the greatest gifts I can bestow on my children."

As Laura's story illustrates, despite the challenges of being a working mom, working outside the home often enriches mothers' lives. According to a 2012 study by Adrianne Frech of the University of Akron and Sarah Damaske of Pennsylvania State University, mothers who work full-time are happier and healthier than mothers who stay at home, work part-time, or are frequently unemployed. The longitudinal study revealed that, of 2,540 women who became mothers between 1978 and 1995, those who went back to work full-time shortly after giving birth reported better physical and mental health than those who did not go back to work full-time. The full-time working moms claimed to have more energy and mobility, and less tendency to depression, at age forty.

On a plane ride in 2012, I sat next to a woman who was pregnant and also had a two year old. After three weeks of staying home with her baby, she noticed that her energy was low; she wasn't herself, and she felt that a piece of her was missing. When she was called in to work during her maternity leave to attend a meeting, as soon as she sat down in the conference room and listened to the buzz of her colleagues, she knew that this was what was missing—she needed to go back to work.

She explained, "It is really about how you are wired. I was never the kind of person who liked to be at home. I like to be out, experiencing life, doing different things and interacting with different people. Work is a huge part of who I am and it really doesn't even feel like work, it is just what I do. It is my passion. I am a happier person when I do what I love, and therefore I am a happier and better mom. But of course there is some amount of guilt. You just can't have it all. You just have to figure out what works for you, in your personal situation. What your childcare options are, what your relationship is with your partner."

Many mothers I surveyed echoed these sentiments; they believe that the happiness, fulfillment, sense of purpose, and balance they derive from working outweigh the downsides, such as not being able to go on many class field trips or make it to all of their child's games or performances. These women know themselves, are connected to their needs, and are comfortable with their choices.

I find work to be beneficial financially and mentally. I need something to be working on outside of the home. And if I can ensure my child receives the care and education that I might not be able to provide as a stay-at-home-mother, then why shouldn't I work and my child attend daycare/preschool? It makes it difficult to complete housework while having a 40-hour/week job, but I manage. It helps to find appreciation in small things, like enjoying a glass of wine and a chunk of cheddar cheese, or a swing on the tree swing after work.
—*MOTHER OF A THREE-YEAR-OLD*

I find working extremely rewarding and it has helped balance my life. Being home for 15 weeks when I had each of my children was great but I missed my adult professional time. My husband and I both work full time, 4 days a week. We have a great balance and do not see any challenges with our current situation.
—*MOTHER OF TWO CHILDREN,*
ages two and eight months

Work is my happy place. Work is the place I can actually accomplish something in its entirety. Home life is never done. There is always something that needs to be done.

Work is who I am. It defines me and I truly enjoy it.
—MOTHER OF THREE CHILDREN,
ages ten, nine, and two

Yet many working women struggle with ambivalence, and also face scrutiny from society and their own children. Although research has shown that society's views about the necessity of women staying home to care for their children has evolved, plenty of people (35 percent of Americans) still assert that a mother's place should be in the home, raising her children and keeping the household running smoothly. And if this pressure is not enough for working moms to question themselves, the children of working moms are not always very understanding or forgiving about cutting them slack regarding their work-related commitments: *Really, Mom, you can't get out of your meeting at work today to come to the dress rehearsal for our school play? I do have a lead role, and all the other moms will be there.*

Another very important way for all moms to care for themselves in regard to their employment choice is to show nonjudgmental compassion toward one another. Leslie Morgan illuminates the unfortunate issue of moms judging other moms for their work choices in her book *Mommy Wars*, in which twenty-six moms—both working and stay-at-home—reveal what their lives are really like, in order to provide moms a better understanding that SAHM is not a code word for eating bonbons all day, and that working moms actually do enjoy spending time with their kids. But Morgan acknowledges that the issue goes much deeper than a mother's employment choice: "The tension between working and at-home moms IS real. But the worst mommy war is the one that rages inside each mom's head as she struggles to feel good about being a mom—no matter what her choices about work. This inner battle plays out on an external stage—through judgments about other moms."[42] So let's all agree to give each other the benefit of the doubt, cut each other some slack, and find out what we can learn from one another, how we can support each other, and how we can help one another find peace with our employment situations.

There is no easy answer for moms when it comes to this important and complicated issue. So many elements come into play, including women's views of themselves, as well as the way in which society views the roles of mothers and fathers in the workplace and at home. Sheryl Sandberg weighs in on this topic in her book *Lean In: Women, Work, and the Will to Lead*: "I believe women can lead more in the workplace. I believe men can contribute more in the home. And I believe that this will create a better world, one where half our institutions are run by women and half our homes are run by men."[43]

◆ ◆ ◆

As grateful as I am to have had time at home with my children, I have two confessions. Confession #1 is that I have always felt pangs of envy toward women who work full-time. Confession #2 is that I question whether or not I could pull it off. Would I be happier and more fulfilled if I got up and went to work every day, instead of trying to manage a bunch of part-time gigs (paid and unpaid) and being overly available to my children? I don't know. But I do believe that whether you are working full-time or part-time or not currently working outside the home, it is essential for you, as part of your self-care solution, to find acceptance of where you are and to trust that you are doing the best you can for yourself and your family. It is also important to remind yourself that if you are not comfortable with your current situation (whether you are working but don't want to be, or you are not working but want to be), you can take the reins of your life by finding happiness in your current situation without giving up on your dreams for the future.

Through research and my many interviews with full-time working mothers (as well as countless hours spent talking with my best friend Laura, who is a full-time working mom with two children), the following is a list of suggestions to help moms manage the work-home juggling act.

SELF-CARE TOOLS FOR MOMS WHO WORK OUTSIDE THE HOME

◆ Let go of guilt. According to Cathy L. Greenberg, Ph.D., and Barrett S. Avigdor, J.D., the authors of the book *What Happy Working Mothers Know*, "Guilt is the enemy of happiness. It is a useless energy waster! Yes, working mothers can have a guilt-free work and life—but it's a choice. Knowing what you truly stand for—understanding your values and sticking to them—[is] what underlie[s] your 'guilt-free life.' You have to make sure you believe in your values and make decisions based on those key values for you—not anyone else."[44]

◆ Assert the value of your work. One working mom of two adult children told me about a time when her young son was crying and hanging on to her foot as she was trying to leave for work one morning. She asked her son, "Do you want to see Mickey Mouse?" Her son nodded through his tears. She replied, "Then please let go of my leg so Mommy can go to work and make the money it will take for us to go to Disney World and see Mickey." He immediately let go of her leg. It is important to help your kids understand the value of your work, whether it is a financial or fulfillment value or both, so they can develop an appreciation and respect for what you do, instead of just looking at it as something that takes you away from them.

◆ Communicate with your family. Explain to your children early on that you will not be able to attend every performance or every game of theirs, and that it is not because you do not care about them or do not want to watch them play or perform (although admittedly, T-ball games and dance recitals can be extremely painful), but that you have work responsibilities that sometimes have to take priority.

It is good for children to know that they are not always the center of Mom's attention and that work is a way for Mom to take care of herself and take care of her family. Also, make sure they understand that they will need to pitch in with housework and other responsibilities so that the house can run smoothly.

◆ Communicate with your partner. Many happy working moms claim that having strong support and good communication with their partners is the key to their ability to feel successful as a mother and an employee or employer. Talk about the division of responsibilities: childcare, cooking, cleaning. Working parents need to continually and clearly communicate with each other about who is doing what, when, and where.

◆ Advocate for yourself at work. As a working mom, you will need a certain amount of flexibility. Make sure to maintain good communication with your superiors and let them know well in advance when you will need to rearrange your schedule for child-related events.

◆ Make time to practice self-care solutions one through five. Exercise, eat right, get enough sleep, and nurture relationships with your partner, friends, and children.

◆ Try to separate work and home life so that when you are home with your family you can focus on spending quality, uninterrupted time with them. When possible, plan fun things to do with your family when you do have time off from work.

◆ Manage your time well. All the working moms I know are incredibly savvy with time management. They grocery shop at lunch, they work through lunch so they can leave an hour early when they need to get to their son's five p.m. baseball game, and they schedule date nights with their partners. Organizational tools such as family calendars can also help with time management and with making sure all family members are aware of each other's commitments.

◆ Let go of perfectionism. The same working mom of two adult children mentioned above told me that her secret to being a happy full-time working mom was that she had a "high tolerance for chaos." In other words, she didn't "sweat the small stuff." The ability to let things go is pivotal to being able to balance work and motherhood (which is probably why I have a difficult time with it). Knowing that you are doing your best to keep all your ducks in a row has to be good enough. Perfection cannot be the goal or you will always be disappointed about some aspect of your life. There are times when things will be running smoothly and then boom, things at work will blow up, or you'll find out that one of your kids is in trouble at school, or your car, your furnace, and your washing machine will all go haywire on the same day. Knowing that there will be bumps and flare-ups as you continually strive for a work-life balance will make you more resilient and better prepared to adapt when the train moves slightly (or significantly) off track.

STAYING HOME WITH YOUR CHILDREN

As author Ayelet Waldman writes in her memoir *Bad Mother*:

> *One day I simply packed up my desk, tossed my framed diplomas into the attic, and became a stay-at-home mom.*
>
> *It was everything I thought it would be. Mommy & Me, story time at the library, Gymboree, long stroller rides with my stay-at-home mommy friends. And then the next day it was Mommy & Me, story time at the library, Gymboree, long stroller rides with my stay-at-home mommy friends. And the day after that, and the day after that, and the day after that. Within a week I had gone mad.*

I took certain satisfaction in the fact that I was now the most important person in the day-to-day life of my child, but I was also bored and miserable. And the fact that I was bored and miserable terrified me. A Good Mother is never bored, is she? She is never miserable. [45]

Raising a family is an ongoing process for working moms and SAHMs alike. But when you stay home with your children, as many SAHMs reveal (and as I have experienced), there are times when you feel like you are in the movie *Groundhog Day*. And as much fulfillment as SAHMs derive from being able to spend invaluable time with their children and see them grow and develop minute by minute, many SAHMs feel that the most challenging aspect of being home with children, especially young children, is that there is no finished product, no sense of completion. There are moments when we think, *Today was a really good day—I am doing a really good job, my baby is thriving, she rolled over, I pumped eight ounces of breast milk and finished three loads of laundry*, but evening comes and it is not time to turn in your completed project to your boss, pack up your briefcase, and head out the door. You look around your house, where you have been most of the day (and have sometimes felt trapped), and you see more dirty dishes, more dirty clothes, and more toys strewn about, and you know that in three hours, you will need to do another feeding and another diaper change.

Raising children is a noble cause. It is a job that is unlike any other job you have had or ever will have. There is no shame in making motherhood your life's work. However, you need to be very honest with yourself in terms of your own fulfillment. If you do feel fulfilled and balanced in this role, then walk proud. But if you don't, there is no need to plaster a fake smile on your face and walk around saying how "completely blessed" you are to be able to be a SAHM. This façade won't work for long. It will come out in all sorts of negative ways, the most common of which is resentment toward your children or your partner, and that will only lead to bitchy mom–bitchy wife syndrome. And I have seen other career-driven moms, who become stay-at-home moms by choice, attempt to fill themselves up with a variety of ultimately empty pursuits: frequent shopping binges that need to be hidden from husbands and which can lead to financial and relational problems; turning to alcohol, food, or drugs to find comfort from the sometimes mundane and isolated world of being a stay-at-home mom; filling social calendars up to the last available minute and becoming engulfed in desperate-housewife drama on a day-to-day basis—once again seeking to fill the void and find purpose outside of poopy diapers and making your own baby food.

Finally, there are the tiger moms who throw themselves into their children's lives with a vengeance, ignoring any and all boundaries; they find themselves in catfights with other moms (*Dance Moms*, anyone?) and battles with teachers and coaches and anyone else who poses a threat to their beloved "star" child, thereby putting an insane amount of pressure on their children.

Regardless of where you are in terms of defining your purpose as a stay-at-home mom, it is essential to be aware when you commit yourself fully and completely to your children that there is no guarantee that, just because you have devoted eighteen years of your life to your child, it doesn't mean he is going to turn out "perfect." For your own self-preservation, you need to be careful that you are not wholly attached to the "outcome" of your child-rearing work, since there are just too many variables. In an effort to ensure that your self-esteem is not completely tied to how your child is faring in life, it is often helpful to have something of your own, unrelated to your children, to balance out your need to feel successful and fulfilled. Even if it is something small, like taking an art class or volunteering for a cause you are passionate about, it can do the trick. Ensuring that you are feeding your own soul will help you be better equipped to feed the souls who are counting on you.

While many moms have mixed feelings about staying home with their children, most express a profound sense of gratitude and fulfillment in being able to stay home and care for their children full time.

Work is work. I have sacrificed my career to become the primary caregiver in our family. While it has been a lengthy and stressful process I am finally at peace knowing I am doing exactly what I am supposed to be doing right now. The rest of it will take care of itself.

—MOTHER OF TWO CHILDREN,
ages fifteen and eleven

I have the same job, 24/7. There is no ride home for me to decompress from the day, my scenery never changes, and I get very little adult contact during the day. However, I'm rewarded with knowing that my children are in the very best possible care I can put them in, and I will have so many memories with them to cherish when they're older.

—MOTHER OF TWO CHILDREN,
ages two and five months

The lack of the extra income is the most challenging for me. The sacrifices we have to make. But the knowledge that I am the one at home when they come home from school. I am the one who takes care of them when they are sick or hurt. Just seeing their smiles and hearing their laughter—I wouldn't change it for anything.

—MOTHER OF SIX CHILDREN,
ages fifteen, twelve, eight (twins), five, and two

The challenges are that you feel alone quite a bit. You miss having adult interaction and there is a lot of pressure on you to make sure you are making right decisions. The reward is knowing that I am with my kids all day, no one else. We also have a special bond that I know we wouldn't have if I worked outside the home.

—MOTHER OF THREE CHILDREN,
ages five, three, and two

On the flip side, many SAHMs grapple with the following questions:

- How do you validate yourself as a SAHM?
- How do you maintain your sense of self when you spend the majority of your day taking care of others?
- How do you find fulfillment in your role as a mother? How do you find fulfillment outside of this role?
- Do you feel valued by your partner? Do you feel like an equal partner?

Without getting regular pats on the back for a "job well done" or a paycheck with your name on it that you can hold up and say, "See, my work is worth something," it can be very difficult for moms to feel respected in their role. A mother with two children, ages ten and fourteen, explained to me how she met her husband while they were both working on Wall Street. "I had the same job as he did and I was making the same amount of money," she explained. "But as soon as I left my job to stay home with our first child, who is special needs, my husband viewed me differently. It became my job not only to serve our child but to serve him. And because he brings home the big paycheck and I don't, I am no longer an equal in his mind. The interesting thing is that I know how to do his job. I did his job and got paid for it. But there is no way he could do my job now. No way. He wouldn't last a day."

Getting on the same page with your partner about each one of your roles, responsibilities, and contributions to the family is an essential component of self-care for SAHMs. Some of the biggest issues and most intense arguments that my husband and I have had over the years have been about the division of home- and kid-related responsibilities. Because he is the breadwinner, does that mean that he gets to leave his dishes in the sink? Hmmm . . . not quite seeing the correlation there; to me, it's as simple as what you learn in kindergarten—clean up after yourself. Although that is obviously a hot button for me, I know I am not alone—this type of issue regarding stereotypical gender roles comes up for many couples as they try to define their individual and collective roles.

> *It is hard. We made the decision together that I would stay home. I am lucky I can do it. I said I would cook, clean, etc. because I am home. But there is a fine line. I am not a housekeeper. If I wanted to be I would have found a paying job. So I have some resentment about that. It is rewarding when I see how well behaved my children are and I know I had a part in that. It is rewarding to see them excel. It is rewarding every day when I get a hug and told that they love me. I love my kids. I do feel sometimes that I just don't get a break. My husband has the pressure of earning the money, and sometimes I feel that is what he respects. I don't contribute to the household moneywise. So that can be a challenge.*
>
> —*MOTHER OF THREE CHILDREN,*
> *ages thirteen, eight, and five*

Furthermore, some mothers express that not only do they feel somewhat undervalued by their partners, they also feel judged by other family members and society as a whole for staying home with their children. SAHMs have to endure publicly critical comments like that of Democratic strategist Hillary Rosen, who stated that Ann Romney, mother of five boys, "has never worked a day in her life."[46]

In the same vein, one mother of three children, ages ten, eight, and six, reveals,

I was surrounded by sisters-in-law who each have big jobs and continued to get bigger and bigger promotions and become more and more successful in their jobs. I was the only stay-at-home-mom on my husband's side of the family and that was not well respected. I felt like my mother-in-law looked down upon me, especially when my kids went back to school. I felt like they thought I did nothing; that I was wasting my education, [my] doctorate degree and my earning potential by staying home. My own mother, however, was glad I was staying home with my kids and didn't think it was a waste at all. And most importantly, I loved it.

A mother of an eleven-year-old similarly describes how she felt judged and undervalued when she stayed at home with her child:

> *When my daughter was born, I stayed home with her for a while, but it was not a good thing for me. Whenever I bought anything, which was not very often, my husband questioned me. My mother-in-law even told me that since I was not making any money, I should not buy anything for myself. I felt useless, dependent, and controlled. I ended up going back to work part time.*

Every one of the stay-at-home moms I have interviewed shares internal and external struggles. And just as it is the case for working moms, being a SAHM requires sacrifices and compromises. There may be days when you wish you could replace your snot-covered sweatshirt with a crisp clean blouse, drop off your child at daycare, and head to work, where you sit at your own quiet, neatly organized desk and scan a to-do list that does not include "feed, burp, change" every few hours. And yet, on the day your son takes his first step or says "Mama" for the first time, or you teach your daughter how to write her name, you may thank G-d that you were able to be home to witness the milestone first hand. There is no question that being a SAHM can be rewarding, but in order to feel good in this role, you must make self-care a part of your everyday life. The following tips will help you find balance, fulfillment, and happiness as a SAHM:

SELF-CARE TOOLS FOR SAHMS

- ◆ Communicate: Talk to your partner about expectations and responsibilities. Talk about what it means to each one of you to have an equal partnership and what this looks like, given that one person is making money and one isn't.

- ◆ Make time to practice self-care solutions one through five. Exercise, eat right, get enough sleep, set boundaries, and nurture relationships with your partner, friends and children.

- ◆ Ask for help. Many SAHMs feel like it is wrong to ask for help with childcare or household responsibilities. It is not wrong. If you can afford some cleaning help, and this allows you to be less stressed and to spend more quality time with your children or quality time taking care of yourself, then get it. If you can afford a babysitter or nanny to help you manage the kid juggling, or you have a family member who is willing to help you out once in a while, say yes to help! Just because you are a SAHM does not mean you have to be rearing children and cleaning your house 24/7.

- ◆ Connect with other SAHMs. Join a playgroup or a mom's group so you have a support network in your community with whom you have regular social interaction, which is essential for SAHMs.

- ◆ Find the joy. As you try to set a feeding, eating, and sleeping schedule for your children, don't be a slave to it. It is okay to shake things up every now and then. Say yes to a lunch date with an old friend and be okay with your baby taking her nap in her car seat for that day, or say yes to an impromptu walk with a neighbor even though it's your child's lunchtime. He can eat Cheerios in the stroller until you get home and feed him lunch.

- ◆ Get out of the house. Just do it. As much of a pain as it is to prepare the bottomless pit of a diaper bag, and to get you and your children dressed and pottied and fed, getting out of your house regularly is pivotal to your sanity and to combat the feeling of being trapped or isolated. Go to the zoo, the park, the museum, meet friends for a picnic, take a walk. Staying active and stimulated is a must for SAHMs.

◆ Cut yourself some slack. An interesting fact: according to a 2014 report by D'vera Cohn, Gretchen Livingston, and Wendy Wang of the Pew Research Center, "Despite the additional time they spend on child care, mothers who do not work outside the home give themselves slightly lower ratings than working mothers for the job they are doing as parents. In a 2012 survey, 66% of stay-at-home mothers rated themselves as 'excellent' or 'very good' parents, compared with 78% of working mothers."[47] This information could be interpreted to mean that SAHMs judge themselves more critically than working moms, which I have seen to be the case. When you are in the trenches with your kids all day long, it can be difficult to keep things in perspective and to be able to step back and say, "Oh, I am doing such a fantastic job as a mother." But, just as it is important for working moms to let go of the guilt of not being with their children all the time, if you are a SAHM, it is key for you to acknowledge that even though you are doing a great job mothering your children, your kids will have bad days, and you will have bad days too.

IS THERE A HAPPY MEDIUM?

According to the above-mentioned report by Cohn, Livingston and Wang, "a plurality of working and stay-at-home mothers said that the ideal situation for them is to work part time. Only 36% of stay-at-home mothers said that not working at all is ideal for them."[48] For me, working part-time has been my salvation.

Not only has it provided me with paychecks (albeit very, very small ones, but nonetheless, with my name on the payee line) and the feeling of making a contribution outside of being a mom, but my part-time work has also helped me maintain a sense of balance. And I was fortunate that most often, I could work my writing and teaching hours around my kids' schedules, which has been key to my ability to balance work and home. The following mothers have also found that working part-time provides them with purpose and flexibility, and they claim that this really is the happy medium:

> *I love what I do and I am passionate about what I do.*
> *I truly enjoy my work and it's only part time so I'm able*
> *to be home with my kids most of the time. I'm grateful*
> *I don't have to choose too often between work and home.*
> *I seem to find an okay balance between what I do outside*
> *of the home and what I do at home.*
>
> —*MOTHER OF TWO CHILDREN,*
> *ages eight and six*

> *I work part-time because that works for me and my*
> *family. It allows me the flexibility and space I need to*
> *be the kind of person, wife, and mother I want to be.*
> *Yes, a larger income would be nice and my husband does*
> *carry much of our financial burden, but what we lose in*
> *money, we gain in peace of mind. To me, an organized,*
> *good flowing home is worth all the money in the world!*
>
> —*MOTHER OF THIRTEEN-YEAR-OLD TWINS*

> *[Work is] a nice escape to adulthood while being a*
> *stay-at-home mom and the primary caretaker. It's nice*
> *to have a part-time job that I love and that allows me*
> *to find balance between mom, individual and woman.*
> *[My husband and I] both work together and take turns*
> *with the baby. Sometimes we're both tired and it's*

*hard to figure things out immediately . . . time and
rest help that! A strong family, lots of communication
and giving each other time to rest/play/breathe/be is
very important.*

—MOTHER OF A TWO-YEAR-OLD

While working part-time can seem like the magic balance for
many women—depending upon the type of part-time work a
mother does and how her work is structured—other moms claim
that working part-time can be more complicated and difficult. In
fact, many moms who work part-time talk about how they put
in way more hours than they get paid for and are continually
frustrated by this. Working Moms expert Katherine Lewis asserts:

*Part time jobs can end up being a trap, where you lose
the respect and advancement of a full-time position,
earn less money and end up working almost as many
hours as your 40-hour-a-week counterparts. . . . One
of the biggest complaints of part time working moms
is that they don't fit in with the working moms and
they don't fit in with the stay-at-home moms. Yes, you
do have more free time, but that doesn't mean you can
volunteer for every school project and chaperone every
field trip. You still have job responsibilities—and likely
more child care duties than the average working mom.
On the other hand, you may catch resentful glances
from full-time working mothers who assume that your
life is easy and stress-free.[49]*

I can relate to this wholeheartedly, as I struggle with
protecting my time to write and meet deadlines, but sometimes
I do feel guilty when I say no to volunteer requests—or even
requests from my kids, which we now know is a boundary issue.
While working part-time does seem to be a good compromise
for me and for many mothers, it is not without its challenges.

SELF-CARE TOOLS FOR
MOMS WHO WORK PART-TIME

- ◆ It is okay to say no. Determine how much more you can take on outside of work and childcare, in terms of managing your son's soccer team, chairing a community fundraiser, or volunteering at your kids' school. Be honest with yourself about your limits and be secure about staying within them.
- ◆ Communicate clearly with your employer about expectations, hours, and pay. If you feel that you are putting in significantly more time than you are being paid for then talk to your supervisor. Do not allow yourself to be taken advantage of.
- ◆ Try to set clear boundaries around work and home so that you can be present with your family and present with your work. This can take a lot of creativity and discipline, but thoughtful planning and strong time management are key.
- ◆ Understand that it is nearly impossible to do it all, and it is certainly impossible to do it all perfectly. Sometimes your work will overwhelm you and need more time and attention, and sometimes your family will require more of you. Cut yourself some slack and trust that you are doing the best you can in managing home, work, and taking care of yourself.
- ◆ Practice self-care tools one through five.

The most important part of the motherhood-work conundrum is not to try to figure out the fail-safe formula—because, as this chapter demonstrates (and as you've most likely experienced), there isn't one. What is certain is that, regardless of whether you are a full-time stay-at-home mom, a full-time working mom, or somewhere in between, you must take care of yourself. Working moms can say they don't have time to exercise just as honestly as SAHMs can. And the truth is, most moms do not have a whole lot of spare time hanging around. But in order to be true to themselves and to stay healthy in their bodies and minds, moms need to *make* time for self-care. Being intentional about self-care will help you to be more present in your work life and your family life, and help you feel better overall so that you can experience more joy in all aspects of your life.

CHAPTER 10:

Self-Care Solution #8—
Never Give Up

"'Taking care of myself is a big job, no wonder why
I avoided it for so long.'"

—*Melody Beattie*, Codependent No More

Attempting to wrap up this book with a neatly tied bow is a near-impossible task because the practice of self-care continually evolves as both you and your kids grow and change. No matter how focused you are on practicing self-care, there will most certainly be times when you feel as if you can't care for yourself the way you want to and know that you need to, and as if you just want to throw in the towel and let yourself go. You are too tired, too stressed, too depressed, too overwhelmed, too overweight, too out of shape, too unmotivated, too "far gone."

But the moment you became a mother, you took both the obvious oath—to care for your child—and another oath, which you may have missed in the frenzy of giving birth (or maybe you were sleeping when the oath-taker came by your hospital room): the promise to take care of yourself so you could take care of your family for as long as you possibly could. While moms don't need to remind themselves to take care of their children, they do need to remind themselves continually to take care of themselves—especially when life gets hard, relationships become challenging, work gets stressful, loved ones become ill, or your children struggle. These are the times when all of the self-care solutions in this book lead up to this last, and perhaps most important one: never give up.

You are the foundation of your family and a pillar of strength for your children, even when you don't feel that strong. And you have a big job to do. As Judith Viorst asserts, women are the managers of the family, which includes being the manager of their children and, oftentimes, of the relationship with their partners. The only way moms can uphold their managerial positions with strength and compassion is to continue to cultivate those traits within themselves, and doing so requires an ongoing, never-give-up commitment to self-care. It is important to believe in yourself, and in your ability to mother your children and to handle whatever obstacles might come their way or your way. But it will be hard—really hard, hard in ways that you could not have imagined. The depth of pain, worry, and fear that mothers carry for and about their children can be almost unbearable at times, even when you are doing your best to take the advice provided in the boundaries chapter. But as my wise rabbi has told me, "G-d gives you what you are capable of handling."

It won't always feel like you are capable of handling your life, your decisions, your kids, your spouse, your parents, or your in-laws, but when you reach into the self-care toolbox that you have now created, you will remember that, even when your tools do not seem to be working and you feel that you are unable to handle certain challenges, the catch-all tool that is always available to you is *never to give up.*

One important thing to remember when you feel as if you are at the end of your rope—physically, mentally or emotionally—is that you are never alone. There are moms all over your community and all over the world who may be experiencing similar challenges. When you feel as if you have reached an insurmountable obstacle within yourself or with your children, reach out to those other mothers, or to your partner, or to anyone who will hold your hand and remind you to stay strong, that you are doing the best you can, and to hang in there. Also remind yourself that it is also okay to express to your children that you are not infallible and that you are not Supermom. As kids get older and develop a better understanding of the human condition, it's okay for you to let them know if you are having a hard time, that you feel overwhelmed, and that you need them to step up a bit and pitch in more to take some of the stress off you.

As devoted to self-care as I have been for my adult life, and certainly throughout the writing of this book, I have been surprised by the number of times I have felt like I've slipped off the self-care track. Yes, I exercise, eat well, and drink plenty of water, but as I have entered into the twilight zone of "mental pause" —otherwise known as menopause—I have needed to add new self-care strategies that, even as of the writing of this book, I am still figuring out.

I have taken trips to the doctor to help me understand why I am "losing my mind" as my body undergoes "the change"; trips to the eye doctor to help me deal with the fact that my vision, like my mind, is becoming blurry; trips to the skin doctor to find out that the dark, "you have a smudge of chocolate on your cheek" spots I've developed are *just* sun spots (oh yeah, like the ones I saw on my grandmother and assured myself that I would *never* have!). I examine the dark circles and lines under my eyes that glare back at me as I look in the bathroom mirror, even before I put my reading glasses on and even after a good night's sleep.

These ongoing changes serve as continual reminders of the fact that my youth is slipping away, no matter how much water I drink. They remind me of how much less energy (and sometimes patience and attention) I have to mother my ten-year-old today than I had to mother my now-twenty-year-old when she was ten.

Then, to add gasoline to my internal fire of emotion, I look around and see mom friends and acquaintances who are battling and sometimes losing battles to diseases, physical and mental; I see moms I care about working jobs that they hate, struggling to make ends meet, caring for (and losing) aging parents, existing in marriages that drain them, and caring for kids who are not well, physically or mentally; I see moms who are trying to heal from the never-ending pain of losing a child. I look at my own battles and the ways in which I am challenged to the core with managing my anxiety, time and time again, as I parent four kids at four very different life stages. The overwhelmed, panic-stricken feeling that I described at the beginning of the book, which led me to melt down at my sister's doorstep, continues to visit me from time to time. I find myself derailed and detached from myself, focusing almost every ounce of available energy I have on my children, family, and others—worrying, racing, running, doing, serving, giving, and meeting others' needs—and thereby sending my own needs downriver. Making no time for my friends, for fun, for my husband, for yoga, writing, or time to myself. Nope, no time for self-care.

But then, as the gas light comes on and exhaustion consumes me, I become irritable with my kids or husband, or I feel like I am on the verge of tears (or, better yet, I have a good cry), and I realize that I am running on empty and that a self-care reboot is in order. Sitting down at my computer, I have gratefully made my way back to this book, rereading chapters and writing new ones, and finding renewed energy, as I have reminded myself that part of not ever giving up means that:

- ◆ It is okay to make mistakes with my children and not feel like a failure.
- ◆ I need to step back from the flurry of life's demands to feel my feelings and not bottle them up inside.
- ◆ I can acknowledge my children's happiness and sadness without carrying their baggage around as if it were my own.
- ◆ It's okay to be confused about approaching middle age and all that goes along with that—looking back, looking forward, while trying to stay focused on the now—needing and wanting to be present and engaged in my life, in my work, and with my ten- and thirteen-year-olds at home, while still parenting two kids away at college on opposite sides of the country.
- ◆ Despite all of the many, many blessings in my life,

which I try to count as often as I can, it is not easy, this motherhood thing. I truly had no idea how hard it would be. And the idea of "bigger kids, bigger problems" is absolutely true.

◆ With each new challenge I face, and in trying to embrace the joy in my life, I wind up right here, utilizing one, two, or ten of the self-care strategies outlined in this book, reminding myself never to give up.

◆ Even when mothers are unable to do the self-care biggies, as much as they would like to (like going to the gym or going out with their partner or girlfriends), we must give ourselves credit for even small acts of self-care:

- *Take a walk to the mailbox by yourself and notice the nature around you.*
- *Give a homeless man a dollar because it feels good to give and because it reminds you that you have a home and that you and your children are not going hungry today.*
- *Take an extra long shower.*
- *Take deep cleansing breaths when you are driving your kids to their activities and silently (or audibly... your kids will find this very amusing) repeat positive messages to yourself like, "I am breathing in self-care, and exhaling stress and negativity."*

On a walk with my husband days before this manuscript was due to the publisher, I was trying to figure out the most important self-care takeaways I wanted to leave readers with as they conclude this book. Here is what we came up with:

◆ The opposite of making yourself a priority is *not* making your kids less of a priority.

◆ Your family's wants cannot be placed above your

needs (which is why you need to be clear on what your needs are).

- ◆ It is your job to fulfill your children's needs, not their wants.
- ◆ And finally, as I've repeated throughout this book, there is no better gift you can give to yourself and your children than the gift of practicing self-care. Your ongoing commitment to maintaining a healthy mind, body, and spirit will enhance not only your life, but your children's as well, teeing them up for a lifetime of practicing their own self-care.

Now that you're equipped with a renewed sense of perseverance and with the enthusiasm of self-care, honor it by recommitting to that oath you made the day your child was born.

> *I, [insert name], promise to take care of myself so that I can take good care of my family. I will not give up on myself as I will not give up on my family. I will teach my children the value of practicing self-care by showing them how it is done through example.*

And every day you can fill in the answer to this question:

> *This is what I am going to do to take care of myself today:_____.*

> *Your signature:*

Period. End of discussion. But really it's only the beginning.

Epilogue

"Letting go doesn't mean we don't care. Letting go doesn't mean we shut down. Letting go means we stop trying to force outcomes and make people behave. It means we give up resistance to the way things are, for the moment. It means we stop trying to do the impossible—controlling that which we cannot—and instead, focus on what is possible—which usually means taking care of ourselves. And we do this in gentleness, kindness, and love, as much as possible."

—*Melody Beattie*, More Language of Letting Go

Confession: I have been "writing a book" for seventeen years. My first attempt began after my oldest son (who is graduating high school in June 2015, as I finish writing this book) had a bout with infant colic and I wanted to offer moms some sort of a survival guide for dealing with colicky babies. I partnered with my dear friend Amy Susman-Stillman and wrote, researched, and interviewed other moms. We even secured an agent who was able to put our proposal in front of some big-name publishers. But another book on colic written by a leading colic expert also landed on their desks right around the same time, and our book got pushed to the side.

As we were deciding on next steps, I became pregnant with my fourth child and my life took a slightly different turn than planned, and the book was tabled. But the process was not all for nothing. Amy and I were able to extract some of the material and publish a few magazine articles about colic; we helped some friends who had colicky babies and learned a great deal about the book-publishing world. And probably the most valuable aspect was that Amy and I stayed in regular, close contact during some of our very difficult first years of parenting.

The next book project, as I mentioned in the introduction, began several years later when I was working for a local parenting magazine called *Momtalk*. *Raising Mom* and *Expect the Unexpected: The Best-Kept Secrets of Modern Motherhood* were a couple of the title contenders. For this project, I was lucky enough to have another friend of mine, Helene Bolter, join me, while Amy stayed in the wings as a consultant.

Helene and I began working together on this tell-all book for moms, hitting every stage of motherhood and discussing some of the surprises, challenges, and joys of each age and stage. But, as I mentioned, while I learned a great deal about mothering through the various stages, and the book proposal sparked the attention of a few publishers, the initial feedback was that the scope was too broad. Once again, I felt a bit deflated by the process, got busy with other commitments, and decided to give my book-writing quest a rest. The book lay dormant in my Mac (it is still there, if anyone is interested in reading it). I shifted gears a bit and enrolled in yoga teacher training, began teaching yoga, and started my blog, *Unscripted Mom*, and Helene went back to work as a child psychologist.

But just as I knew I wasn't finished having children after my second child, I knew I was not finished with this book project. Despite the fact that I was continually pulled off focus by the demands of my family, part-time work, and volunteer commitments that I had a difficult time saying no to, I continued to believe that something very important was evolving from all my research, interviews, surveys, and life experiences. It gnawed at me. It would not leave me alone.

Finally, after poring over the surveys time and time again and realizing what truly resonated with me, the self-care theme hit me over the head. But while I knew then that self-care would be the focus of the book, what I didn't realize was how much self-care *I* would need to practice to complete this book.

In talking to two local writer friends, Galit Breen and Kate Hopper—who have written books while caring for young children and working full- or part-time—I learned about their writing process. They told me that for a certain amount of time, while zeroing in on getting their books done, they did only what was absolutely necessary for their families in order to stay focused on their goal at hand. They were disciplined and committed to their projects and communicated this to their friends and loved ones, and they asked for the physical and moral support they needed—self-care and self-advocacy at its finest. In addition to the fact that I truly needed to practice what I preached in order to finish this book, I also realized that in my almost two decades of studying moms and their relationships with themselves and with their families, I have repeatedly seen that self-care is the key to dealing with almost any issue that a mom will face.

Writing this book required me to look closely at the ways in which I do and do not practice self-care, and what works and what doesn't. I also believe that it helped me to become a better mother—better not in terms of "perfect," but better as in more accepting of myself, my strengths, my weaknesses, and my blind spots. My hope is that every mother who reads it will find this to be true for her as well.

Writing this book was also hard. Really hard. And scary. There were many times along the way when I truly did not think I had it in me to finish. I had already left two books unfinished, unpublished. Maybe this would just be one more to add to the pile. Plus, it was painful to write this book, to be honest with myself in opening old wounds that sometimes I could not get to heal.

"I can't do it," I told my therapist during a session in March 2015. "I can't finish it."

"Why?"

"I am too scared," I told her through tears.

"What is scary about finishing your book?" she prodded.

With a deep sigh, I realized that the ever-too-familiar feelings of shame and self-doubt, which I thought I had successfully evicted, had crept back into my psyche. "Because I reveal things about myself that I have not revealed publicly and I am afraid people will judge me. And I am afraid the book will fail, that no one will buy it, that I don't have what it takes to sell it, that I will hate it once it's published and I won't be able to change it. Nope, I can't do it. I just can't."

"This book is *you*," she said gently. "This book is about acceptance and vulnerability and letting go. You need to believe that you are good enough, with your flaws, with your mistakes. You need to trust that your voice is strong and important, and that you and the other moms in this book deserve to be heard and that your sharing of your experiences will provide strength to other moms. You need to stay committed to believing in yourself so you can finish this book and publish it. And then you need to let it go," she said gently. "Finishing the book and allowing others to read it is your self-care."

There it was again. I knew it, I wrote it, I believed it, and yet I was still scared out of my mind. More self-care was needed. So I turned to family and friends, who provided me with great doses of support and encouragement. I leaned on my amazing editor, Annie Tucker, who assured me that almost every author she has worked with reaches that point of fear and panic as the book gets closer to completion. As hard as I tried to push all of that negativity away and win the bet that I had with my high school senior (the same son that was the impetus for my "first book" on infant colic) who said I wouldn't finish my book before he graduated, I did not win. But I came close, and that bet did give me the necessary, ongoing kick in the butt to take this book all the way to the finish line. So, in the spirit of self-care, I set a bunch of self-doubting baggage and fear aside and decided to go with Sheryl Sandberg's advice, from her book *Lean In: Women, Work and the Will to Lead*: "Done is better than perfect."[50] Here I am in June of 2015 writing the conclusion of the book, three weeks after his high school graduation.

As much as I wish I could report that I have completely mastered self-care after nearly four years of dissecting it, that would be a bit of a stretch. I don't think that anyone necessarily masters self-care, just as no one masters yoga (or parenting). It is a practice. What I can say, however, is that the awareness I have gained from this process truly has been life-changing. It has forced me to continue to dig deeper, to be more in touch with my needs and the needs of others. I have learned how to better separate all of the needs, and healthily manage both. I have learned that self-care and self-advocacy do not equate to selfishness, and that neglecting myself to care for others is not a sustainable program.

Writing this book has given me the strength to own my story, thereby releasing me from far too much shame. During the time I have been writing this book, I wrote a piece in *Brain, Child* magazine about the first time I told my seventeen-year-old daughter about my eating disorder and how I thought that would destroy her respect for me and damage our relationship. While our relationship did change after I relayed my struggle to her, it actually changed for the better. She had a deeper understanding of me and ultimately showed more compassion toward me. In October of 2014, I co-led a workshop on self-care at a Twin Cities Jewish Community Conference on Mental Health, and in February 2015, during National Eating Disorders Awareness week, I was a guest on a local radio show and shared my experience with listeners across the state. And my work as a volunteer at the Emily Program has also allowed me to share my story of struggle and survival with parents and caregivers of children, teens and young adults who are suffering from eating disorders and the anxiety and depression that often accompanies the disease.

Implementing the self-care strategies in this book has strengthened my relationships with my children, my husband, and my friends—but most of all, with myself. Fighting a life-and-death battle with self-care was a terrifying experience and it has taken me a long time to find solid ground. And my journey continues, as every single day I still have to ask myself what self-care means to me today. My hope is that after reading this book, you will habitually ask yourself the same question, and that self-care won't be something that you "will get to when . . . "

The time for self-care is now. Embrace yourself. Embrace your self-care so that you can continue to nurture and expand your heart every day in order for you to share your love with those you love.

Acknowledgements

The process of writing this book has spanned two decades and has involved far too many people to name, yet they have all directly or indirectly influenced my understanding and application of self-care, and I am grateful to each and every one of them. There are several people who I need to recognize for their unwavering support and encouragement, and for their pivotal role in the completion of this book.

To Nina Badzin, thank you for becoming my first true writer friend, welcoming me into the local and national writing and blogging community, teaching me the tricks of the trade, and trudging through the writing trenches with me, spinning rejections into opportunities and celebrating any and all victories, no matter how small. To my friend, local editor, and beam of positivity, Kate Hopper, I am grateful for you. And to the many other wonderful Twin Cities and national writers and thinkers who have inspired me with their writing, their ideas, and their kindness and support, this book would not be what it is without your influence—Lisa Barr, Lee Wolfe Blum, Helaine Bolter, Susan Bonne, Galit Breen, Ashley Davis Bush, Emily Mitty Cappo, Betsy Conway, Nate Garvis, Gran Harlow, Mary Dell Harrington, Hilary Levey Friedman, Jordana Green, Lisa Heffernan, Michelle Millar, Lynn Nelson, Daisy Pellant, Tammie Rosenbloom, Rox Sandovsky and the Friday writing gang, Michelle Segar, Jessica Smock, Jill Smokler, Marcelle Soviero, Stephanie Sprenger, Denny Stockdale, Amy Susman-Stillman, Gary Swartz, and The Twin Cities Writing Studio group members—thank you all! Thank you to Professor Tom Conley, my first writing mentor, who told me at age 21, "Julie, if you can *think*, you can *write*." Those words continue to inspire me every day.

To the wonderful, masterful creators of books at She Writes Press—Brooke Warner, Katherine Sharpe, and Lauren

Wise, thank you for diligently guiding me through this process. It has been a pleasure to work with such talented and creative women. And to my editor Annie Tucker, whose keen insight, word mastery, honesty, guidance, and kind heart took my words and ideas and helped me craft them into this book. I could not have done this without you, my friend.

Thank you to Amber, Brenda, Dan, Debi, Erika, Holly, Jane, Julz, Rabbi K, Lauren, LB, Lisa, Sandra, Sara, Sydney, Trissa, Tzeporah Leah, Vico, Wendy, my book club and Torah study members, CPY Minnetonka, and the Breck School community for enriching my life and my children's lives. To my rocks, who knew me when, and know me now and always, Dina and Laura . . . thank g-d for you. To Lisa, Malka, and Rebecca, you are everywhere in this book, and in my heart. I am forever grateful for your kindness, insight, and care.

To my wonderful family, the Monros, and the whole Soskin/Becker/Lurie gang—my mentors, friends, teachers, and spoilers of my children, thank you. Joy, thank you for always reading my work and for your invaluable feedback. Dan, Abigail, Ben, Dee, Harlan, and Mom B., I am grateful for the love. To Nick, Emi and ZZ (and Zoe)—I couldn't ask for better. Mom and Dad, thank you for believing in me and for your generous hearts. Natalie, my sister, my best friend, the yin to my yang, "thank you" does not begin to cover it.

To Sophie, Jeremy, Abe, and Josie, thank you for the incredible gift of being your mother, for filling my heart with love, joy, and happiness, for the lessons you teach me every day (even the tough ones), and for making me laugh harder than anyone in the world (except for Dad…sometimes). And here you go, JG, it is really done.

And to the love of my life—David, I am eternally grateful for the magical, passionate, everlasting love we share, and for the incredible family we have created. Being your partner is a true blessing. YAMTC.

BIBLIOGRAPHY

Achor, Shawn. *The Happiness Advantage: The Seven Principles of Positive Psychology That Fuel Success and Performance at Work*. New York: Broadway Books, 2010.

Adams, Thelma. "Do I Have Enough Fun?" *O, the Oprah Magazine*. February, 2015, 91.

Arnold-Ratliff, Katie. "Do I Feel My Feelings?" *O, the Oprah Magazine*, February, 2015, 94.

Beattie, Melody. *The Language of Letting Go*. Center City: Hazelden, 1990.

Benton, Sarah. "Caron Study Reveals 'Top 5 Reasons' Mothers Turn to Alcohol." *Psychology Today* (blog), May 10, 2013. https://www.psychologytoday.com/blog/the-high-functioning-alcoholic/201305/caron-study-reveals-top-5-reasons-mothers-turn-alcohol.

Berkner, Laurie. "Balancing Work and Motherhood." *Huffington Post*, October 10, 2012. http://www.huffingtonpost.com/laurie-berkner/work-life-balance-song_b_1937106.html.

Brooks, Kim. "Is Motherhood Causing My Depression?" *Salon.com*, February 25, 2013. http://www.salon.com/2013/02/25/is_motherhood_causing_my_depression/.

Brown, Brene', *I Thought It Was Just Me (but it isn't): Making the Journey from "What Will People Think?" to "I Am Enough"*. New York: Gotham Books, 2008.

Bryner, Jeanna. "Even Preschool Girls Favor Being Thin, Study Finds." *Live Science*, November 16, 2010. http://www.livescience.com/8984-preschool-girls-favor-thin-study-finds.html.

Buehler, Cheryl, and Deborah P. Welsh. "A process model of adolescents' triangulation into parents' marital conflict: The role of emotional reactivity." *Journal of Family Psychology* 23, no. 2 (April 2009): 167–80.

Bush, Ashley Davis and Daniel Arthur Bush. *75 Habits For a Happy Marriage—Marriage Advice to Recharge and Reconnect Every Day*. Avon, MA: Adams Media, 2013.

Carlson, Richard. *Don't Sweat the Small Stuff—and It's All Small Stuff: Simple Ways to Keep the Little Things from Taking over Your Life*. New York: Hyperion, 1997.

Cettina, Teri. "The Secret to a Stronger Marriage." *Parenting.com*, accessed August 26, 2015. http://www.parenting.com/article/the-secret-to-a-stronger-marriage.

Cohn, D'Vera, Gretchen Livingston, and Wendy Wang. "After Decades of Decline, A Rise in Stay-at Home Mothers." Washington, D.C.: Pew Research Center's Social & Demographic Trends project, April 2014.

Davis, Eraina. "Mommy Wars: My Interview With Leslie Morgan Steiner." *ChicagoNow*, August 17, 2015. http://www.chicagonow.com/the-good-life/2015/08/mommy-wars-my-interview-with-leslie-morgan-steiner/.

Ephron, Nora. *Heartburn*. New York: Knopf, 1983.

Emmons, Robert. *Gratitude Works!: A Twenty-one-day Program for Creating Emotional Prosperity*. San Francisco: Jossey Bass, 2013.

———. "How Gratitude Can Help You Through Hard Times." *The Greater Good Science Center*, May 13, 2013. http://greatergood.berkeley.edu/article/item/how_gratitude_can_help_you_through_hard_times.

Field, Alison E., et. al. "Weight Concerns and Weight Control Behaviors of Adolescents and Their Mothers." *Archives of Pediatrics and Adolescent Medicine* 159, no. 12 (2005): 1121-1126.

Frech, Adrianne, and Sarah Damaske. "The Relationships between Mothers' Work Pathways and Physical and Mental Health." *Journal of Health and Social Behavior* 53, no. 4 (2012): 396–412.

Lewis, Katherine. "The Top 5 Cons of Part-Time Jobs." *About.com Parenting*, accessed August 26, 2015. http://workingmoms.about.com/od/workschedule/a/5-Cons-Of-Part-Time-Jobs.htm.

"Get the Facts on Eating Disorders." *National Eating Disorders Association*, accessed August 25, 2015. http://www.nationaleatingdisorders.org/get-facts-eating-disorders.

"Giving Thanks Can Make you Happier." *Harvard Health Publications*, November, 2011. http://www.health.harvard.edu/healthbeat/giving-thanks-can-make-you-happier.

Goldsmith, Barton. *Emotional Fitness for Intimacy: Sweeten & Deepen Your Love in Only 10 Minutes a Day*. Oakland, CA: New Harbinger Publications, 2009.

———. "The Difference Between Sex and Intimacy." *Psychology Today* (blog), September 30, 2013. https://www.psychologytoday.com/blog/emotional-fitness/201309/the-difference-between-sex-and-intimacy.

Greenberg, Cathy, and Barrett S. Avigdor. *What Happy Working Mothers Know: How New Findings in Positive Psychology Can Lead to a Healthy and Happy Work/Life Balance*. Hoboken: John Wiley & Sons, 2009.

Harriger, Jennifer A., et. al., "Body Size Stereotyping and Internalization of the Thin Ideal in Preschool Girls." *Sex Roles* 63, no. 9-10: 609-620.

Ivy, John, "Why Breakfast Is the Most Important Meal of the Day." *EAS Academy*, accessed August 25, 2015. http://easacademy.org/trainer-resources/article/why-breakfast-is-the-most-important-meal-of-the-day-eas-academy

Kashdan, Todd B. "The Parent's Balance Sheet." *Psychology Today*, October, 2012, 52.

Knepper, Cheryl. *Women and The Impact of Addiction: Special Issues in Treatment and Recovery*. Caron Treatment Centers. Accessed August 27, 2015. https://www.naatp.org/wp-content/uploads/2012/07/Knepper-Women-Presentation.pdf.

Kucinich, Jackie, and Martha T. Moore. "Hilary Rosen says Ann Romney never worked 'day in her life'" *USA Today*, April 12, 2012. http://usatoday30.usatoday.com/news/politics/story/2012-04-12/ann-romney-hilary-rosen-work/54235706/1.

Lahey, Jessica. "Students Aren't Getting Enough Sleep—School Starts Too Early." *TheAtlantic.com*, Aug. 25, 2014. http://www.theatlantic.com/education/archive/2014/08/surprise-students-arent-getting-enough-sleep/379020/.

Lifland, Shari. "Advice for Working Moms: Get Happy!" *American Management Association*, last modified August 14, 2014. http://www.amanet.org/training/articles/Advice-for-Working-Moms-Get-Happy.aspx.

Lino, Mark. *Expenditures on Children by Families, 2013*. Alexandria: US Department of Agriculture, Center for Nutrition Policy and Promotion, 2014. http://www.cnpp.usda.gov/sites/default/files/expenditures_on_children_by_families/crc2013.pdf.

Maxon, Seth. "How Sleep Deprivation Decays the Mind and Body." *The Atlantic.com*, Dec. 30, 2013. http://www.theatlantic.com/health/archive/2013/12/how-sleep-deprivation-decays-the-mind-and-body/282395/.

Mayo Clinic Staff. "Exercise: 7 benefits of regular physical activity." *The Mayo Clinic*, accessed August 26, 2015. http://www.mayoclinic.org/healthy-lifestyle/fitness/in-depth/exercise/art-20048389.

McGhee, Paul. "Humor and Health." *HolisticOnline.com*. Accessed August 26, 2015. http://www.holistic-online.com/humor_therapy/humor_mcghee_article.htm.

Miller, Karen Maezen. *Momma Zen: Walking the Crooked Path of Motherhood*. Boston: Shambhala, 2006.

Mogel, Wendy. *The Blessing of a Skinned Knee: Using Jewish Teachings to Raise Self-reliant Children*. New York: Scribner, 2008. First published 2001 by Simon & Schuster.

National Heart, Lung and Blood Institute. "How Much Sleep Is Enough?" Last updated February 22, 2012. https://www.nhlbi.nih.gov/health/health-topics/topics/sdd/howmuch.

National Sleep Foundation. "Teens and Sleep." Accessed August 27, 2015. http://sleepfoundation.org/sleep-topics/teens-and-sleep.

———. *2014 Sleep in America Poll: Sleep in the Modern Family.* Alexandria, VA: National Sleep Foundation. Accessed August 25, 2015. http://sleepfoundation.org/sites/default/files/2014-NSF-Sleep-in-America-poll-summary-of-findings---FINAL-Updated-3-26-14-.pdf

NBC and AOL. "TODAY/AOL Ideal To Real Body Image Survey." *AOL.* February, 2014. http://www.aol.com/article/2014/02/24/loveyourselfie/20836450/.

O'Connor, Anahad. "Really? Using a Computer Before Bed Can Disrupt Sleep." *Well* (blog), *The New York Times,* September 10, 2012. http://well.blogs.nytimes.com/2012/09/10/really-using-a-computer-before-bed-can-disrupt-sleep/?_r=0.

Paddock, Catharine. "Working Moms Enjoy Better Physical And Mental Health." *Medical News Today,* August 22, 2012.

Paul, Jordan and Margaret Paul. *Do I Have to Give up Me to Be Loved by You?* Center City, MN: Hazelden, 2002.

Paul, Margaret. "Are You an Enmeshed Parent?" *World of Psychology* (blog), *Psychcentral.com.* Accessed August 26, 2015. http://psychcentral.com/blog/archives/2012/07/05/are-you-an-enmeshed-parent/.

Pawlowski, A. "Hitting the Mommy Juice Too Hard? Experts Warn of Alcohol Abuse by Moms." *TODAY Parents,* April 2014. http://www.today.com/parents/hitting-mommy-juice-too-hard-experts-warn-alcohol-abuse-moms-2D79473508.

Pogrebin, Letty Cottin. "Golda Meir." *Jewish Women: A Comprehensive Historical Encyclopedia, Jewish Women's Archive.* March 20, 2009. http://jwa.org/encyclopedia/article/meir-golda.

Quindlen, Anna. *Loud and Clear.* New York: Random House, 2004.

Raffelock, Dean, and Robert Roundtree. *A Natural Guide to Pregnancy and Postpartum Health.* New York: Avery, 2003.

Rizzo, Kathryn M., Holly H. Schiffrin, and Miriam Lis. "Insight into the Parenthood Paradox: Mental Health Outcomes of Intensive Mothering." *Journal of Child and Family Studies* 22, no. 5 (2013): 614-620.

Rosemond, John K. *John Rosemond's New Parent Power!* Kansas City, MO: Andrews McMeel, 2001.

Ross, Carolyn Coker. "Why Do Women Hate Their Bodies?" *World of Psychology* (blog), *Psychcentral.com*. June 2, 2012. http://psychcentral.com/blog/archives/2012/06/02/why-do-women-hate-their-bodies/.

Rubin, Gretchen. *The Happiness Project: Or Why I Spent a Year Trying to Sing in the Morning, Clean My Closets, Fight Right, Read Aristotle, and Generally Have More Fun.* New York, NY: Harper, 2009.

Rutten, Geert M., et. al., "Interrupting long periods of sitting: good STUFF." *International Journal of Behavioral Nutrition and Physical Activity* 10, no. 1 (2013). doi:10.1186/1479-5868-10-1.

Sandberg, Sheryl, and Nell Scovell. *Lean In: Women, Work, and the Will to Lead.* New York: Alfred A. Knopf, 2013.

Sapirstein, Milton R. *Emotional Security.* New York: Crown, 1948.

Sholl, Jessie. "Shutting Shame Down." *Experience Life.com*. October, 2013. https://experiencelife.com/article/shutting-shame-down/.

Singhal, Anupriya. "Moms May Influence Children's Body Image." *The Harvard Crimson*, December 14, 2005. http://www.thecrimson.com/article/2005/12/14/moms-may-influence-childrens-body-image/.

Smock, Jessica, and Stephanie Sprenger. *The HerStories Project: Women Explore the Joy, Pain, and Power of Female Friendship.* CreateSpace Independent Publishing Platform, 2013.

Steiner, Leslie Morgan. *Mommy Wars: Stay-at-home and Career Moms Face off on Their Choices, Their Lives, Their Families.* New York: Random House, 2006.

Tartakovsky, Margarita. "Self-Care Strategies for Busy Moms. " *World of Psychology* (blog), *Pyschcentral*. May 1, 2014. http://psychcentral.com/blog/archives/2014/01/05/self-care-strategies-for-busy-moms/.

Tiemann, Amy. *Mojo Mom: Nurturing Your Self While Raising a Family.* New York: Penguin, 2009.

Wade, T. D., A. Keski-Rahkonen, and J. Hudson. "Epidemiology of eating disorders." In *Textbook in Psychiatric Epidemiology, 3rd Ed.*, edited by M. Tsuang and M. Tohen, 343-360. New York: Wiley, 2011.

Waldman, Ayelet. *Bad Mother: A Chronicle of Maternal Crimes, Minor Calamities, and Occasional Moments of Grace.* New York: Doubleday, 2009.

Walton, Alice. "The Better Mother? How Intense Parenting Leads to Depression." *Forbes.com*, July 6, 2012. http://www.forbes.com/sites/alicegwalton/2012/07/06/the-better-mother-how-intense-parenting-leads-to-depression/.

"What is Depression." *National Institute of Mental Health*. Accessed August 26, 2015. https://www.nimh.nih.gov/health/topics/depression/index.shtml.

Williams, Mary Elizabeth. "We're Clean Eating Our Way to New Eating Disorders." *Salon.com*, January 15, 2015. http://www.salon.com/topic/eating_disorders/.

Wood, B., et. al. "Light level and duration of exposure determine the impact of self-luminous tablets on melatonin suppression." *Applied Ergonomics* 44, no. 2 (March 2013): 237-40.

SELF-CARE RESOURCE LIST
SUGGESTED READING

EXERCISE AND NUTRITION

Billis, Stacie. *One Hungry Mama*. http://onehungrymama.com/.

Fed Up. Dir. Michele Simon. Weinstein Company, 2014.

Food, Inc. Dir. Robert Kenner. Magnolia Home Entertainment, 2009.

Freytag, Chris. *Get Healthy U*. http://gethealthyu.com/.

Hello Healthy. http://blog.myfitnesspal.com/.

Jamieson, Alexandra. *Women, Food, and Desire: Embrace Your Cravings, Make Peace with Food, Reclaim Your Body*. New York: Gallery Books, 2015.

McGruther, Jenny. *Nourished Kitchen*. http://nourishedkitchen.com/.

Segar, Michelle L. *No Sweat: How the Simple Science of Motivation Can Bring You a Lifetime of Fitness*. New York: AMACOM, 2015.

Wachob, Jason. *mindbodygreen*. http://www.mindbodygreen.com/.

FRIENDSHIP

Dobransky, Paul, and L. A. Stamford. *The Power of Female Friendship: How Your Circle of Friends Shapes Your Life*. New York: Penguin, 2008.

Lerner, Harriet Goldhor. *The Dance of Connection: How to Talk to Someone When You're Mad, Hurt, Scared, Frustrated, Insulted, Betrayed, or Desperate*. New York: HarperCollins, 2001.

Smock, Jessica, and Stephanie Sprenger. *The HerStories Project: Women Explore the Joy, Pain, and Power of Female Friendship*. CreateSpace Independent Publishing Platform, 2013.

Sonnenberg, Susanna. *She Matters: A Life in Friendships*. New York: Scribner, 2013.

Vernon, Mark. *The Meaning of Friendship*. New York: Palgrave Macmillan, 2010.

GRATITUDE/HAPPINESS

Achor, Shawn. *The Happiness Advantage: The Seven Principles of Positive Psychology That Fuel Success and Performance at Work*. New York: Broadway Books, 2010.

Gillespie, Becky Beaupre, and Hollee Schwartz Temple. *Good Enough Is the New Perfect: Finding Happiness and Success in Modern Motherhood*. Don Mills, Ont.: Harlequin, 2011.

Hanson, Rick. *Hardwiring Happiness: The New Brain Science of Contentment, Calm, and Confidence*. New York: Crown Publishing, 2013.

Kaplan, Janice. *The Gratitude Diaries: How a Year Looking on the Bright Side Can Transform Your Life*. New York: Penguin, 2015.

Martin, Rachel. *Finding Joy*. http://www.findingjoy.net/.

Quindlen, Anna. *A Short Guide to a Happy Life*. New York: Random House, 2000.

Rubin, Gretchen. *The Happiness Project: Or Why I Spent a Year Trying to Sing in the Morning, Clean My Closets, Fight Right, Read Aristotle, and Generally Have More Fun*. New York: HarperCollins, 2009.

———. *Better than Before: Mastering the Habits of Our Everyday Lives*. New York: Crown, 2015.

Wachob, Jason. *Q & A with Kris Carr: Crazy Sexy Inspirational Wellness Rock Star*. Mindbodygreen. June 28, 2010. http://www.mindbodygreen.com/0-1024/Q-A-with-Kris-Carr-Crazy-Sexy-Inspirational-Wellness-Rock-Star.html.

Meditation/Spirituality/Yoga

Adele, Deborah. *The Yamas and Niyamas: Exploring Yoga's Ethical Practice*. Duluth, MN: On-Word Bound Books, 2009.

Gates, Rolf, and Katrina Kenison. *Meditations from the Mat: Daily Reflections on the Path of Yoga*. New York: Anchor, 2002.

Headspace, Inc. *Headspace*. https://www.headspace.com/.

Lasater, Judith. *Living Your Yoga: Finding the Spiritual in Everyday Life*. Berkeley, CA.: Rodmell Press, 2000.

Telushkin, Joseph. *The Ten Commandments of Character: Essential Advice for Living an Honorable, Ethical, Honest Life*. New York: Bell Tower, 2003.

Motherhood/Parenting

Bronson, Po, and Ashley Merryman. *NurtureShock: New Thinking about Children*. New York: Twelve, 2009.

Brown, Brené, *The Gifts of Imperfect Parenting: Raising Children with Courage, Compassion, and Connection*. Louisville, CO: Sounds True, 2013. Audiobook.

Haims, Julie. *How to Raise an Adult: Break Free of the Overparenting Trap and Prepare Your Kid for Success*. New York: Henry Holt and Company, 2015.

Harrington, Mary Dell, and Lisa Heffernan. *Grown and Flown*. http://grownandflown.com/.

Mogel, Wendy. *The Blessing of a Skinned Knee: Using Jewish Teachings to Raise Self-reliant Children*. New York: Scribner, 2001.

Mogel, Wendy. *The Blessing of a B Minus: Using Jewish Teachings to Raise Resilient Teenagers*. New York: Scribner, 2010.

Naumburg, Carla. *Parenting in the Present Moment: How to Stay Focused on What Really Matters*. Berkeley: Parallax Press, 2014.

Rotbart, Harley. *No Regrets Parenting: Turning Long Days and Short Years into Cherished Moments with Your Kids*. Kansas City, MO.: Andrews McMeel, 2012.

Stafford, Rachel Macy. *Hands Free Mama*. http://www.handsfreemama.com/.

Smokler, Jill. *Scary Mommy: A Parenting Community for Imperfect Parents*. https://www.scarymommy.com/.

Soviero, Marcelle. *Brain, Child—The Magazine for Thinking Mothers*. http://www.brainchildmag.com/.

Tiemann, Amy. *Courageous Parents, Confident Kids: Letting Go So You Both Can Grow*. Chapel Hill: Spark Press, 2010.

PERSONAL GROWTH

Brown, Brené. Any and all books, CDs, or TED Talks.

Chavis, Sibyl. *The Possibility of Today*. http://www.possibilityoftoday.com/.

Gilbert, Elizabeth. Big Magic: *Creative Living Beyond Fear*. New York: Riverhead Books, 2015.

Melton, Glennon Doyle. *Carry On, Warrior: The Power of Embracing Your Messy, Beautiful Life*. New York: Scribner, 2013.

Neff, Kristin. *Self-Compassion Step by Step: The Proven Power of Being Kind to Yourself*. Louisville, CO: Sounds True, 2013. Audiobook.

Neff, Kristin. *Self-Compassion: Stop Beating Yourself Up and Leave Insecurity Behind*. New York: William Morrow, 2011.

Oettingen, Gabriele. *Rethinking Positive Thinking: Inside the New Science of Motivation*. New York: Penguin, 2014.

Relationship with Spouse/Partner

Bush, Ashley Davis and Daniel Arthur Bush. *75 Habits For a Happy Marriage—Marriage Advice to Recharge and Reconnect Every Day*. Avon, MA: Adams Media, 2013.

Chapman, Gary. *The 5 Love Languages: The Secret to Love That Lasts*. Chicago: Northfield, 2010.

Doherty, William. *Take Back Your Marriage: Sticking Together in a World That Pulls Us Apart*. 2nd ed. New York: Guilford, 2013.

Gottman, John Mordechai, and Nan Silver. *The Seven Principles for Making Marriage Work*. New York: Crown, 1999.

Johnson, Susan. *Hold Me Tight: Seven Conversations for a Lifetime of Love*. New York: Little, Brown, 2008.

Kerner, Ian, and Heidi Raykeil. *Love in the Time of Colic: The New Parents' Guide to Getting It on Again*. New York: HarperCollins, 2009.

Wachtel, Ellen F. *We Love Each Other, But—: Simple Secrets to Strengthen Your Relationship and Make Love Last*. New York: St. Martin's Griffin, 1999.

Stay-at-Home Moms/Working Moms

Alcorn, Katrina. *Maxed Out: American Moms on the Brink*. Berkeley, CA: Seal, 2013.

Greenberg, Cathy, and Barrett S. Avigdor. *What Happy Working Mothers Know: How New Findings in Positive Psychology Can Lead to a Healthy and Happy Work/Life Balance*. Hoboken, NJ: John Wiley & Sons, 2009.

Sandberg, Sheryl, and Nell Scovell. *Lean In: Women, Work, and the Will to Lead*. New York: Alfred A. Knopf, 2013.

Stanton, Melissa. *The Stay-at-Home Survival Guide: Field-Tested Strategies for Staying Smart, Sane and Connected While Caring for Your Kids*. Berkeley, CA: Seal, 2008.

Steiner, Leslie Morgan. *Mommy Wars: Stay-at-home and Career Moms Face Off On Their Choices, Their Lives, Their Families*. New York: Random House, 2006.

NOTES

Chapter 3:
Self-Care Solution #1—
Honor Your Body

1 Brown, 197.

2 NBC and AOL, 5.

3 Wade, et. al.

4 Harriger

5 Bryner

6 Singhal

7 Sholl

8 Ibid.

9 Mogel, 148.

10 Ibid., 164.

11 Ivy

12 Rutten, et. al.

Chapter 4:
Self-Care Solution #2—
Embrace Sleep and Rest

13 Raffelock, Rountree, Hopkins, and Block, 263.

14 National Sleep Foundation, "Teens and Sleep."

15 Ibid.

16 Lahey

17 Wood, et. al.

18 Rubin, 14

19 Rizzo, Schiffrin, and Lis

20 Adams, 91.

21 Rubin, 147.

22 Ibid., 6.

23 Rizzo, Schiffrin, and Lis

24 National Institute of Mental Health, "What is Depression?"

25 Rizzo, Schiffrin, and Lis

26 Quindlen, 14-15.

Chapter 6:
Self-Care Solution #4—
Find Gratitude and Connection

27 Harvard Health Publications

28 Emmons, "How Gratitude Can Help You Through Hard Times."

29 Beattie, 218.

30 Arnold-Ratliff, 94.

31 Smock and Sprenger, 2.

32 Knepper

33 Benton

34 Pawlowski

Chapter 7:
Self-Care Solution #5—
Set Boundaries

35 Pirkei Avot 1:14

36 Paul, "Are You an Enmeshed Parent?"

Chapter 8:
Self-Care Solution #6—
Nurture Your Partnership

37 Cettina

38 Ibid.

39 Lino

40 Buehler and Welsh

41 Goldsmith, "The Difference Between Sex and Intimacy."

Chapter 9:
Self-Care Solution #7—
Find Work-Life Balance

42 Davis

43 Sandberg, 172.

44 Lifland

45 Waldman, 12.

46 Kucinich and Moore

47 Devara, Livingston, and Wang, 29.

48 Ibid.

49 Lewis

Epilogue

50 Sandberg, 123.

ABOUT THE AUTHOR

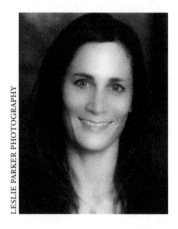

LESLIE PARKER PHOTOGRAPHY

JULIE BURTON is a freelance writer, blogger, co-founder of the Twin Cities Writing Studio, a yoga instructor, a wife of twenty-two years and a mother of four children, ranging in age from twenty-one to eleven. She earned her advanced degree from the Medill School of Journalism at Northwestern University, is the former editor of *Momtalk Magazine*, and writes about parenting, relationships, the aging process, and self-care on her blog juliebburton.com (www.juliebburton.com), as well as on local and national websites and publications. She lives in Minnetonka, Minnesota, with her family.

SELECTED TITLES FROM SHE WRITES PRESS

She Writes Press is an independent publishing company founded to serve women writers everywhere. Visit us at www.shewritespress.com.

Stop Giving it Away: How to Stop Self-Sacrificing and Start Claiming Your Space, Power, and Happiness by Cherilynn Veland. $16.95, 978-1-63152-958-0. An empowering guide designed to help women break free from the trappings of the needs, wants, and whims of other people—and the self-imposed limitations that are keeping them from happiness.

The Thriver's Edge: Seven Keys to Transform the Way You Live, Love, and Lead by Donna Stoneham. $16.95, 978-1-63152-980-1. A "coach in a book" from master executive coach and leadership expert Dr. Donna Stoneham, The Thriver's Edge outlines a practical road map to breaking free of the barriers keeping you from being everything you're capable of being.

Think Better. Live Better. 5 Steps to Create the Life You Deserve by Francine Huss. $16.95, 978-1-938314-66-7. With the help of this guide, readers will learn to cultivate more creative thoughts, realign their mindset, and gain a new perspective on life.

The Complete Enneagram: 27 Paths to Greater Self-Knowledge by Beatrice Chestnut, PhD. $24.95, 978-1-938314-54-4. A comprehensive handbook on using the Enneagram to do the self-work required to reach a higher stage of personal development.

Mothering Through the Darkness: Women Open Up About the Postpartum Experience edited by Stephanie Sprenger and Jessica Smock. $16.95, 978-1-63152-804-0. A collection of thirty powerful essays aimed at spreading awareness and dispelling myths about postpartum depression and perinatal mood disorders.

Learning to Eat Along the Way by Margaret Bendet. $16.95, 978-1-63152-997-9. After interviewing an Indian holy man, newspaper reporter Margaret Bendet follows him in pursuit of enlightenment and ends up facing demons that were inside her all along.